Malignant Pleural Mesothelioma: State of the Art

Editor

BRYAN M. BURT

THORACIC SURGERY CLINICS

www.thoracic.theclinics.com

Consulting Editor
VIRGINIA R. LITLE

November 2020 • Volume 30 • Number 4

ELSEVIER

1600 John F. Kennedy Boulevard • Suite 1800 • Philadelphia, Pennsylvania, 19103-2899

http://www.thoracic.theclinics.com

THORACIC SURGERY CLINICS Volume 30, Number 4
November 2020 ISSN 1547-4127, ISBN-13: 978-0-323-75964-9

Editor: John Vassallo (j.vassallo@elsevier.com)
Developmental Editor: Laura Fisher

Thoracic Surgery Clinics (ISSN 1547-4127) is published quarterly by Elsevier Inc., 360 Park Avenue South, New York, NY 10010-1710. Months of publication are February, May, August, and November. Business and editorial offices: 1600 John F. Kennedy Boulevard, Suite 1800, Philadelphia, PA 19103-2899. Periodicals postage paid at New York, NY, and additional mailing offices. Subscription prices are $393.00 per year (US individuals), $623.00 per year (US institutions), $100.00 per year (US students), $460.00 per year (Canadian individuals), $806.00 per year (Canadian institutions), $100.00 per year (Canadian students), $225.00 per year (international students), $480.00 per year (international individuals), and $806.00 per year (international institu-tions). Foreign air speed delivery is included in all Clinics' subscription prices. All prices are subject to change without notice. **POSTMASTER:** Send address changes to Thoracic Surgery Clinics, Elsevier Health Sciences Division, Subscription Customer Service, 3251 Riverport Lane, Maryland Heights, MO 63043. **Customer Service (orders, claims, online, change of address): Telephone: 1-800-654-2452 (U.S. and Canada); 314-447-8871 (outside U.S. and Canada). Fax: 314-447-8029. E-mail: jour-nalscustomerservice-usa@elsevier.com (for print support); journalsonlinesupport-usa@elsevier.com (for online support).**

Reprints. For copies of 100 or more, of articles in this publication, please contact Commercial Rights Department, Elsevier Inc., 360 Park Avenue South, New York, NY 10010-1710. Tel: 212-633-3874; Fax: 212-633-3820; E-mail: reprints@elsevier.com.

Thoracic Surgery Clinics is covered in *MEDLINE/PubMed (Index Medicus), EMBASE/Excerpta Medica, Science Citation Index Expanded (SciSearch®), Journal Citation Reports/Science Edition,* and *Current Contents®/Clinical Medicine.*

Printed in the United States of America.

Contributors

CONSULTING EDITOR

VIRGINIA R. LITLE, MD
Professor, Department of Surgery, Chief,
Division of Thoracic Surgery, Boston
University, Boston, Massachusetts, USA

EDITOR

BRYAN M. BURT, MD, FACS
Associate Professor and Chief, Division of
Thoracic Surgery, The Michael E. DeBakey
Department of Surgery, Baylor College of
Medicine, Houston, Texas

AUTHORS

MARJAN ALIMI, MD
Department of Cardiothoracic Surgery, NYU
Langone Medical Center, New York, New York,
USA

RAPHAEL BUENO, MD
Chief, Division of Thoracic Surgery, Brigham
and Women's Hospital, Harvard Medical
School, Boston, Massachusetts, USA

MICHELE CARBONE, MD, PhD
Department of Thoracic Oncology, John A.
Burns School of Medicine, University of
Hawaii Cancer Center, Honolulu, Hawaii,
USA

LUCIAN R. CHIRIEAC, MD
Department of Pathology, Brigham and
Women's Hospital, Harvard Medical School,
Boston, Massachusetts, USA

MARC DE PERROT, MD, MSc, FRCSC
Director, Mesothelioma Program, Division of
Thoracic Surgery, University Health Network,
Princess Margaret Cancer Center, Toronto
General Hospital, Toronto, Ontario, Canada

ASSUNTA DE RIENZO, PhD
Investigator, Division of Thoracic Surgery,
Brigham and Women's Hospital, Harvard
Medical School, Boston, Massachusetts, USA

LAURA L. DONAHOE, MD, MSc, FRCSC
Division of Thoracic Surgery, Toronto General
Hospital, Princess Margaret Cancer Center,
University Health Network, Toronto, Canada

CALEB J. EUHUS, MD
Department of Surgery, Division of General
Thoracic Surgery, The Michael E. DeBakey
Department of Surgery, Baylor College of
Medicine, Houston, Texas, USA

RAJA M. FLORES, MD
Ames Professor of Cardiothoracic Surgery,
Chairman, Department of Thoracic Surgery,
Mount Sinai Health System, Icahn School of
Medicine at Mount Sinai, New York, New York,
USA

KATARZYNA FURRER, MD
Attending Physician, Department of Thoracic
Surgery, University Hospital Zurich, Zurich,
Switzerland

CHANDRA M. GOPARAJU, PhD
Senior Scientist, Department of Cardiothoracic Surgery, NYU Langone Medical Center, New York, New York, USA

YIN P. HUNG, MD, PhD
Department of Pathology, Massachusetts General Hospital, Harvard Medical School, Boston, Massachusetts, USA

ISABELLE OPITZ, MD
Director, Department of Thoracic Surgery, University Hospital Zurich, Zurich, Switzerland

HARVEY I. PASS, MD
Stephen E. Banner Professor of Thoracic Oncology, Vice-Chairman, Research, Department of Cardiothoracic Surgery, Director, General Thoracic Surgery, NYU Langone Medical Center, New York, New York, USA

R. TAYLOR RIPLEY, MD
Department of Surgery, Division of General Thoracic Surgery, The Michael E. DeBakey Department of Surgery, Baylor College of Medicine, Houston, Texas, USA

KENNETH E. ROSENZWEIG, MD
Professor and Chair, Department of Radiation Oncology, Icahn School of Medicine at Mount Sinai, New York, New York, USA

KIMBERLY J. SONG, MD
Assistant Professor, Department of Thoracic Surgery, Mount Sinai Health System, Icahn School of Medicine at Mount Sinai, New York, New York, USA

BENJAMIN WADOWSKI, MD
Postdoctoral Fellow, Division of Thoracic Surgery, Brigham and Women's Hospital, Harvard Medical School, Boston, Massachusetts, USA

ANDREA S. WOLF, MD, MPH
Associate Professor, Department of Thoracic Surgery, Director, New York Mesothelioma Program, Mount Sinai Health System, Icahn School of Medicine at Mount Sinai, New York, New York, USA

HAINING YANG, PhD
Department of Thoracic Oncology, John A. Burns School of Medicine, University of Hawaii Cancer Center, Honolulu, Hawaii, USA

Contents

Despite multiple diagnostic toolkits, the diagnosis of diffuse malignant pleural mesothelioma relies primarily on proper histologic assessment. The definitive diagnosis of diffuse malignant pleural mesothelioma is based on the pathologic assessment of tumor tissue, which can be obtained from core biopsy sampling, pleurectomy, or other more extensive resections, such as extrapleural pneumonectomy. Given its rarity and overlapping microscopic features with other conditions, the histologic diagnosis of diffuse malignant pleural mesothelioma is challenging. This review discusses the pathologic features and the differential diagnosis of diffuse malignant pleural mesothelioma, including select diagnostic pitfalls.

Malignant pleural mesothelioma (MPM) is a rare, aggressive malignancy of the pleural lining associated with asbestos exposure in greater than 80% of cases. It is characterized by molecular heterogeneity both between patients and within individual tumors. Next-generation sequencing technology and novel computational techniques have resulted in a greater understanding of the epigenetic, genetic, and transcriptomic hallmarks of MPM. This article reviews these features and discusses the implications of advances in MPM molecular biology in clinical practice.

Malignant pleural mesothelioma (MPM) is an asbestos-related neoplasm that can only be treated successfully when correctly diagnosed and treated early. The asbestos-exposed population is a high-risk group that could benefit from sensitive and specific blood- or tissue-based biomarkers. We review recent work with biomarker development in MPM and literature of the last 20 years on the most promising blood- and tissue-based biomarkers. Proteomic, genomic, and epigenomic platforms are covered. SMRP is the only validated blood-based biomarker with diagnostic, monitoring and prognostic value. To strengthen development and testing of MPM biomarkers, cohorts for validation must be established by enlisting worldwide collaborations.

Staging of malignant pleural mesothelioma has been challenging because of a paucity of cases and poor survival. At least 5 staging systems were proposed before 1990 until the first consensus system was published in 1995. This system used tumor, node, metastasis designations and borrowed heavily from parenchymal lung cancer descriptors. With the establishment of a database to collect cases from 1995 to 2013, evidence-based revisions to the 1995 staging classification were published in 2016. With improving imaging technology, clinical staging will become more refined and, it is hoped, more useful for prognostication even without operative resection.

In the absence of standardized treatment algorithms for patients with malignant pleural mesothelioma, one of the main difficulties remains patient allocation to therapies with potential benefit. This article discusses clinical, radiologic, pathologic, and molecular prognostic factors as well as genetic background leading to preoperative identification of benefit from surgery, which have been investigated over the past years to simplify and at the same time specify patient selection for surgical treatment.

Extended pleurectomy and decortication (ePD) is a difficult operation performed for the surgical resection of malignant pleural mesothelioma that can achieve a macroscopic complete resection with preservation of the lung. With lower perioperative mortality, similar long-term survival, and better tolerance in patients with lower performance status, ePD has become the preferred operation rather than extrapleural pneumonectomy despite lack of a direct comparison. As ePD has become more popular, international collaboration is underway to create surgical guidelines based on collection of operative data. These efforts will improve the safety and standardization of this operation.

Extrapleural pneumonectomy (EPP) is the most extensive form of surgery for mesothelioma, involving en bloc resection of visceral and parietal pleura, lung, diaphragm and pericardium, with reconstruction of the pericardium and diaphragm. It can be performed safely in carefully selected patients. It should be performed in experienced centers as part of a multimodality treatment plan. The SMART approach, with a short course of induction hemithoracic radiation followed by EPP has demonstrated safety and value of hypofractionated hemithoracic radiation combined with complete macroscopic resection. We are conducting a clinical trial with oligofractionated hemithoracic radiation in early-stage mesothelioma.

THORACIC SURGERY CLINICS

THE CLINICS ARE AVAILABLE ONLINE!
Access your subscription at:
www.theclinics.com

Foreword
Malignant Pleural Mesothelioma: An Insidious Disease

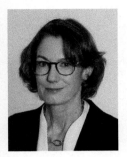

Virginia R. Litle, MD
Consulting Editor

We are excited to bring you this focused issue for the *Thoracic Surgery Clinics* on "Malignant Pleural Mesothelioma," an insidious disease with a projected rise in incidence secondary to environmental factors, including the World Trade Center tragedy, which transpired almost 20 years ago. Our previous issue on this topic was appropriately guest edited by the legendary Dr David Sugarbaker in the inaugural year when *Chest Surgery Clinics* was renamed *Thoracic Surgery Clinics* in 2004. After many advances in the field, including molecular characterization of the tumor, identification of potential biomarkers, and controversies about surgical and multimodality management, a current report was indeed indicated!

As mentored by Dr Sugarbaker from postgraduate training to his leadership position at Baylor, Dr Bryan M. Burt follows in the footsteps of this surgical giant to bring together some of the experts in this field so we may stay abreast of clinical and translational advances in the management of mesothelioma. In the words of one of Dr Sugarbaker's many trainees, we must maintain a "focused attention and clarity of purpose," especially when pursuing and evolving through this increasingly complex world of academic and clinical surgery. Wise words to move our specialty forward and to benefit our patients.

Thank you to our contributors and to guest editor, Dr Burt. May he continue in the footsteps of a thoracic giant—to advance the area of mesothelioma management but also to inspire intellectual curiosity in future generations of thoracic surgeons. We hope you will enjoy this issue!

Virginia R. Litle, MD
Division of Thoracic Surgery
Department of Surgery
Boston University
88 East Newton Street
Collamore Building, Suite 7380
Boston, MA 02118, USA

E-mail address:
Virginia.litle@bmc.org

Twitter: @vlitlemd (V.R. Litle)

Thorac Surg Clin 30 (2020) ix
https://doi.org/10.1016/j.thorsurg.2020.08.009
1547-4127/20/© 2020 Published by Elsevier Inc.

Preface
Malignant Pleural Mesothelioma

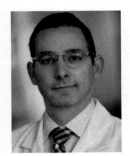

Bryan M. Burt, MD, FACS
Editor

Malignant pleural mesothelioma (MPM) is a highly fatal malignancy of the pleura that has defeated standard-of-care therapy for decades. The most common cause of MPM is industrial/environmental exposure to asbestos in approximately 80% of cases, although it can result from radiation and is occasionally idiopathic. The 3 common histologic subtypes of MPM are epithelial (60%), biphasic (30%), and sarcomatoid (10%), and patients with epithelial MPM generally have better survival than those with nonepithelial histology. Although MPM is a rare disease (0.6% of annual cancer deaths), its worldwide incidence is projected to rise due to continued asbestos exposure from manufacturing, accidents, and abatement. The public health hazard in the United States persists in incidents ranging from asbestos-abatement projects to the September 11, 2001 destruction of the World Trade Center, which exposed millions of individuals to airborne asbestos. Asbestos use is not regulated in most countries, and exposure of Americans and others to asbestos continues via international travel, trade, and military deployments. After a latency period of 15 to 60 years following asbestos exposure, MPM grows rapidly along the parietal and visceral pleura, invades the lung, heart, and mediastinum, and results in death. Surgery is a pillar in the treatment of MPM, and in combination with systemic therapy and/or radiotherapy, extends survival. Because of its unique growth pattern, however, principles of surgery for MPM are unique when compared with most other solid tumors. For example, R0 resection is not possible in MPM, and macroscopic complete resection, an R1 resection, is the objective of surgery for MPM. In this issue of *Thoracic Surgery Clinics*, experts in the field review the state of the art in MPM.

Bryan M. Burt, MD, FACS
Division of Thoracic Surgery
The Michael E. DeBakey Department of Surgery
Baylor College of Medicine
Baylor Clinic
6620 Main Street, Suite 1325
Houston, TX 77030, USA

E-mail address:
Bryan.Burt@bcm.edu

Thorac Surg Clin 30 (2020) xi
https://doi.org/10.1016/j.thorsurg.2020.08.008
1547-4127/20/© 2020 Published by Elsevier Inc.

Pathology of Malignant Pleural Mesothelioma

Yin P. Hung, MD, PhD[a], Lucian R. Chirieac, MD[b],*

KEYWORDS

- Mesothelioma • Pathology • Epithelioid • Biphasic • Sarcomatoid • Immunohistochemistry • BAP1
- Differential diagnosis

KEY POINTS

- Diagnosis of malignant mesothelioma is based on assessment of histologic and immunophenotypic features.
- Classification of malignant mesothelioma (into epithelioid, biphasic, and sarcomatoid types) is based on assessment of cytologic features and has prognostic value.
- A panel of immunohistochemical markers is needed to distinguish sarcomatoid mesothelioma from sarcomatoid carcinoma, sarcomas, and mimics.
- Loss of nuclear BAP1 staining is specific but not sensitive in distinguishing malignant mesothelioma from reactive mesothelial proliferations.
- Correlation with clinical, radiologic, and molecular features is helpful in diagnostic conundrums.

INTRODUCTION

Malignant mesothelioma originates from the cells in the serosal lining that surrounds the body cavities. Of all mesotheliomas, approximately 85% arise from the pleura, approximately 15% arise from the peritoneum, and the remainder (<1%) originates from the pericardium or the tunica vaginalis.[1] In the United States, diffuse malignant pleural mesothelioma affects approximately 3000 patients each year, with an annual incidence of approximately 1 in 100,000.[2,3] Diffuse malignant pleural mesothelioma shows a predilection for men and affects mostly the elderly,[4–6] although the age of distribution is wide, with young patients including adolescents reported.[7] The signs and symptoms can be nonspecific and, depending on the extent of tumor involvement, include pleuritic chest pain, dyspnea, night sweats, and weight loss.[8] Patients with diffuse malignant pleural mesothelioma are managed by trimodality therapy including surgery, chemotherapy, and radiotherapy.[9,10] The use of immunotherapy is under active clinical investigations.[11] The clinical outcome nonetheless remains generally dismal, with a median overall survival of 1 to 2 years.[6] Regarding the pathogenesis of diffuse malignant pleural mesothelioma, a history of asbestos exposure was noted in approximately 70% of patients.[4] Other etiologic factors include exposure to nonasbestos mineral fibers,[12] therapeutic radiation exposure for prior malignancy,[13,14] and in the setting of chronic inflammatory conditions.[15–17] Furthermore, germline alterations in *BAP1* and other tumor suppressors have been implicated in the development of diffuse malignant pleural mesothelioma in a subset of patients.[18,19]

The definitive diagnosis of diffuse malignant pleural mesothelioma is based on the pathologic assessment of tumor tissue, which is obtained from core biopsy sampling, pleurectomy, or other more extensive resections. To establish a pathologic diagnosis of malignant mesothelioma, diagnostic tools that are used clinically include histologic assessment, immunohistochemistry, electron microscopy, cytogenetics, and molecular

a Department of Pathology, Massachusetts General Hospital, Harvard Medical School, 75 Francis Street, Boston, MA 02115, USA; b Department of Pathology, Brigham and Women's Hospital, Harvard Medical School, 75 Francis Street, Boston, MA 02115, USA
* Corresponding author.
E-mail address: lchirieac@bwh.harvard.edu

Thorac Surg Clin 30 (2020) 367–382
https://doi.org/10.1016/j.thorsurg.2020.08.007
1547-4127/20/© 2020 Elsevier Inc. All rights reserved.

techniques (eg, targeted next-generation sequencing, fluorescence in situ hybridization, and single-nucleotide polymorphism arrays). Despite the multiple diagnostic toolkits, the diagnosis of diffuse malignant pleural mesothelioma relies primarily on proper histologic assessment. Given its rarity and overlapping microscopic features with other benign and neoplastic conditions, the histologic diagnosis of diffuse malignant pleural mesothelioma is challenging, with misdiagnoses reported in greater than 60% of cases in some regions in the world as determined by retrospective review.[20] In this review, we discuss the pathologic features and the differential diagnosis of diffuse malignant pleural mesothelioma, including select diagnostic pitfalls.

GROSS FEATURES

Grossly, diffuse malignant pleural mesothelioma presents with circumferential pleural thickening or multifocal-to-diffuse pleural nodules that display a tan-white cut surface (**Fig. 1**A). Invasion into adjacent structures, such as diaphragm, chest wall, pericardium, and interlobular septae of lung, may be seen. In exceptionally rare cases, diffuse malignant pleural mesothelioma presents with diffuse lung parenchymal involvement, with radiographic and gross appearances mimicking an interstitial lung disease.[21]

MICROSCOPIC FEATURES

Diffuse malignant pleural mesothelioma is classified into three histologic types: (1) epithelioid, (2) biphasic (mixed), and (3) sarcomatoid.[1] The determination of histologic types is based on the cytologic features of the tumor. Epithelioid mesothelioma is characterized by epithelioid-to-round cells (**Fig. 1**B, C). Sarcomatoid mesothelioma is characterized by spindled cells with tapered nuclei (**Fig. 1**E, F). Biphasic mesothelioma harbors epithelioid and sarcomatoid components in various proportions, with each comprising at least 10% of the tumor (**Fig. 1**D).

Within each histologic type, diffuse malignant pleural mesothelioma is divided into several subtypes and patterns based on its cytologic, architectural, and background stromal features.[22] In epithelioid mesothelioma, tumor cells are usually epithelioid-to-round; other rare variants include clear cell, signet ring cell, rhabdoid, deciduoid, and small cell.[23–25] Tumor cells are arranged in diverse architectural patterns that include tubulopapillary, trabecular, solid, acinar, micropapillary, or adenomatoid, among others. In sarcomatoid mesothelioma, subtypes described

include conventional/spindle cell, desmoplastic,[26,27] and lymphohistiocytoid.[28–30] A subset of sarcomatoid mesothelioma exhibits heterologous differentiation with osteosarcomatous, chondrosarcomatous, and/or rhabdomyosarcomatous elements.[27]

The assignment of histologic type is challenging, given the intertumoral and intratumoral morphologic heterogeneity. In some cases, it is difficult to distinguish between neoplastic spindled tumor cells (sarcomatoid component) and reactive stromal fibroblasts; the diagnosis of biphasic mesothelioma and epithelioid mesothelioma with prominent stroma is challenging.[31] Furthermore, there is considerable interobserver variability in the recognition of histologic types, even among mesothelioma expert pathologists, with the lowest interobserver agreements in biphasic mesotheliomas.[31–33] Proper type assignment in malignant mesothelioma is nonetheless important, given the prognostic differences among different histologic types. In addition, the accuracy of histologic types varies with the extent of tissue sampling.[34–36] In a study comparing the concordance between histologic types in initial biopsies with subsequent resections, the accuracy of typing increases with a higher number of biopsies.[36] Although sarcomatoid histology in biopsies is highly predictive of sarcomatoid histology in resections, epithelioid histology in biopsies is not entirely specific and is changed to biphasic or sarcomatoid types in resections in up to 20% of patients.[36]

HISTOLOGIC CRITERIA FOR DIFFUSE MALIGNANT PLEURAL MESOTHELIOMA

In diffuse malignant pleural mesothelioma, the goals of histologic assessment are to confirm the pathologic diagnosis and to determine the histologic type, which allows for prognostication and treatment planning. For the diagnosis of diffuse malignant pleural mesothelioma, one needs to establish each of the three conditions discussed next.

The Lesion Is Diffuse and Not Solitary

First, correlation with clinical and radiologic findings is needed to confirm that the distribution of the tumor is diffuse rather than solitary. Although nearly all (>99%) malignant pleural mesotheliomas are diffuse, rare cases of localized pleural mesothelioma have been described, which are solitary, have a different pathogenesis, and harbor a less aggressive clinical course.[37–40]

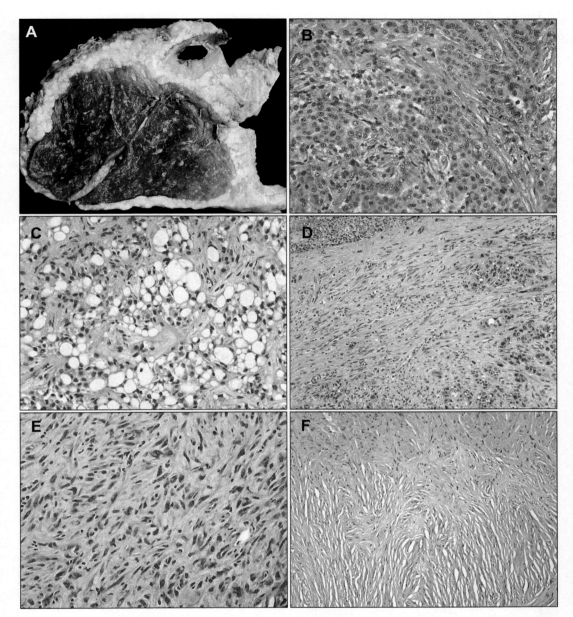

Fig. 1. Gross and histologic features of diffuse malignant pleural mesothelioma. (*A*) Gross photograph of diffuse malignant pleural mesothelioma surrounding lung parenchyma. (*B*) Epithelioid mesothelioma with tubulopapillary pattern. (*C*) Epithelioid mesothelioma with prominent vacuolation, mimicking signet ring cell carcinoma. (*D*) Biphasic mesothelioma, with sarcomatoid and epithelioid components. (*E*) Sarcomatoid mesothelioma. (*F*) Desmoplastic mesothelioma, with tumor cells scattered among storiform fibrosis.

The Lesional Cells Are Mesothelial

Given the morphologic overlap between malignant mesothelioma and diverse mimics, such as carcinomas, immunohistochemistry and, less commonly, electron microscopy is used to confirm the presence of mesothelial differentiation in the tumor cells. Other tools, such

as cytogenetics and molecular analysis, may also be helpful in some instances (discussed later).

The Lesional Cells Are Malignant

Histologic assessment is integral to establish that the mesothelial cells are malignant. Morphologic features that distinguish malignant mesothelioma from reactive conditions (**Fig. 2**) include:

- Invasion into adjacent tissue, such as adipose tissue, skeletal muscle, and lung
- Full-thickness pleural involvement
- Formation of expansile nodules (considered as a type of stromal invasion)

The presence of invasion is considered to be the most reliable criterion in distinguishing malignant mesothelioma from reactive mesothelial proliferations.[41,42] However, such features as necrosis, cytologic atypia, and mitoses should be interpreted with caution, because each are seen in reactive pleuritis and do not necessarily indicate malignancy. Although the diagnosis of malignant mesothelioma can be straightforward when the morphologic features are overly malignant, some cases are challenging: sarcomatoid/desmoplastic mesothelioma may mimic chronic fibrosing pleuritis. Interpretation is difficult when there is limited diagnostic tissue, tangential sectioning, artifacts from histologic processing, and/or entrapment of

adjacent structures mimicking invasion.[41,43] For a mesothelial proliferation that is suspicious for but not definitive for malignancy, one may report the findings as "atypical mesothelial proliferation" and recommend rebiopsy and/or close follow-up. In the distinction between malignant mesothelioma and reactive mesothelial proliferations, the role of ancillary studies had been limited until recently, when BAP1 or MTAP immunohistochemistry and *CDKN2A* copy number assessment by fluorescence in situ hybridization may aid the distinction in some instances (discussed later).

IMMUNOHISTOCHEMICAL FEATURES
Diagnostic Markers to Confirm Mesothelial Differentiation

Immunohistochemistry is integral to the pathologic diagnosis of malignant pleural mesothelioma in clinical practice. Useful immunohistochemical markers include positive markers to confirm mesothelial differentiation, such as WT1, calretinin, and D2-40 (**Fig. 3**A–C); and negative markers to exclude mimics, such as polyclonal CEA, TTF-

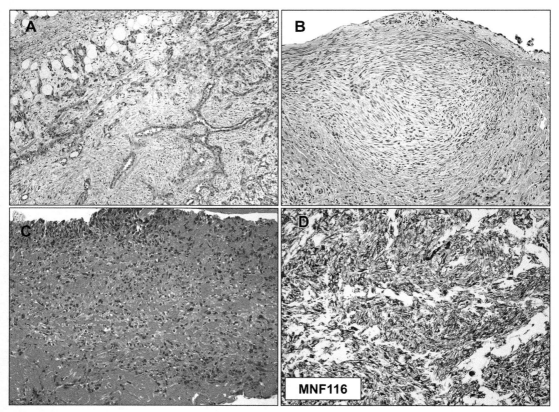

Fig. 2. Diagnostic features of diffuse malignant pleural mesothelioma. (*A*) Invasion into fibroadipose tissue. (*B*) Formation of expansile nodules. (*C*) Lack of zonation with full-thickness involvement. (*D*) Immunohistochemistry for keratin MNF116 in *C* highlights the increased number of tumor cells.

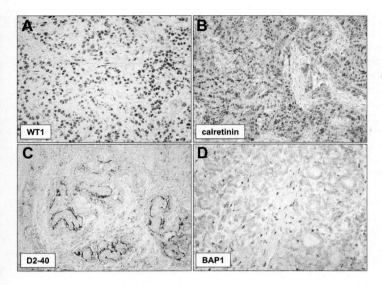

Fig. 3. Immunophenotypic features of diffuse malignant pleural mesothelioma. (*A*) Nuclear WT1 expression. (*B*) Cytoplasmic and nuclear calretinin staining. (*C*) Membranous D2-40 staining. (*D*) Loss of BAP1 nuclear staining.

1, and claudin-4.[44–46] Broad-spectrum keratins are not specific and are expressed in mesotheliomas and carcinomas. Other novel markers recently described include glypican-1 as a positive marker for epithelioid mesothelioma,[47] HEG1 as a positive marker for mesotheliomas,[48,49] and MUC4 as a negative marker,[50,51] although data on their performance in clinical practice remain limited. As one of the caveats, no individual immunohistochemical marker is entirely sensitive and specific. Each of the established mesothelial markers (WT1, calretinin, and D2-40) is expressed in a subset of carcinomas. Conversely, epithelial markers (BerEP4 and MOC31) are expressed in a subset of mesotheliomas, although TTF1 (for adenocarcinoma), p40 (for squamous cell carcinoma), and claudin 4 (for carcinoma)[45] are generally specific although not entirely sensitive. In the guidelines from the International Mesothelioma Panel (MesoPath) and International Mesothelioma Interest Group (iMig), a panel comprising at least two mesothelial markers (calretinin, WT1, D2-40) and two epithelial markers (Claudin 4, TTF1, polyclonal CEA) should be used to establish the diagnosis.[52] In the evaluation of positive markers, the expression of mesothelial markers is focal and limited (especially in sarcomatoid mesothelioma[53]; in fact, there is no consensus on the minimum percentage of cells needed to show marker expression).[54] A 10% staining cutoff has been proposed to be most sensitive and specific in using TTF1 and calretinin immunohistochemistry to distinguish between epithelioid mesothelioma and lung adenocarcinoma,[55] although whether these cutoffs are applicable for other antibodies, histologic

types of mesothelioma, and differential diagnoses remains unclear.

BAP1 (BRCA1-associated protein-1) is a tumor suppressor implicated in the pathogenesis of malignant mesothelioma, uveal melanoma, cholangiocarcinoma, and clear cell renal cell carcinoma.[56] Recurrent somatic and/or germline mutations in *BAP1* are present in malignant mesothelioma. As a surrogate for *BAP1* genomic status, BAP1 immunohistochemistry is used as a diagnostic marker for malignant mesothelioma. Aberrant BAP1 protein expression, defined as complete loss of nuclear BAP1 staining (**Fig. 3**D; including absence of staining or the presence of cytoplasmic BAP1 staining only), is seen in approximately 50% to 70% of diffuse malignant pleural mesothelioma, epithelioid type[57–63] but less than 20% in sarcomatoid type.[64] Aberrant BAP1 expression is seen in 20% of cholangiocarcinoma[65]; 10% of clear cell renal cell carcinoma[66]; and rarely most other carcinomas, including in less than 1% of non–small cell lung carcinomas.[67,68] In diagnostically problematic cases, aberrant BAP1 expression favors malignant mesothelioma and excludes lung carcinoma.[67,68]

Sarcomatoid mesothelioma and sarcomatoid (pleomorphic/spindle cell) carcinoma overlap in their histologic and immunohistochemical features, therefore requiring the use of multiple markers for definitive distinction. Sarcomatoid mesothelioma often shows focal to absent expression for most mesothelial markers, with the most sensitive marker being D2-40/podoplanin.[53,69] Immunohistochemical markers that may aid the distinction between sarcomatoid mesothelioma and sarcomatoid carcinoma include p40 and p63 (for squamous cell carcinoma), TTF1 (for adenocarcinoma), and calretinin (for mesothelioma).[54] Recently, GATA3 has been explored as a potential diagnostic marker for sarcomatoid mesothelioma,[70] with GATA3 expression in only approximately 10% to 20% of non–small cell lung carcinomas[71] including sarcomatoid carcinoma.[70] One can render an accurate diagnosis of sarcomatoid mesothelioma when encountering a spindle/pleomorphic tumor that expresses multiple mesothelial but not epithelial markers; conversely, a diagnosis of carcinoma is made for a sarcomatoid tumor that expresses multiple epithelial but not mesothelial markers. For sarcomatoid tumors that do not show clear-cut mesothelial or epithelial differentiation despite extensive immunohistochemistry work-up, one may not render a definitive diagnosis.[54] In these instances, correlation with clinical, radiologic, and molecular findings may be helpful.[27]

Diagnostic Markers to Confirm a Malignant Mesothelial Proliferation

Although the distinction between malignant mesothelioma and reactive mesothelial proliferations primarily relies on histologic assessment, this is challenging in some cases. Immunohistochemical markers, such as glucose transporter-1 (GLUT1), insulin-like growth factor II mRNA binding protein 3 (IMP3), epithelial membrane antigen (EMA), desmin, and p53, have been explored over the years as potential diagnostic adjuncts. Because they are not entirely sensitive or specific, their utility to distinguish malignant mesothelioma from reactive proliferations on a case-by-case basis is limited.[72,73]

BAP1 immunohistochemistry is a specific (although not sensitive) marker to distinguish malignant mesothelioma from reactive mesothelial proliferations. Aberrant BAP1 expression (complete loss of staining or cytoplasmic staining only) is seen in approximately 50% to 70% of diffuse malignant pleural mesothelioma[57–63]; whereas, reactive proliferations show intact BAP1 nuclear staining.[57,58,61,63] In particular, the utility of BAP1 to distinguish sarcomatoid mesothelioma from reactive pleuritis is limited, because BAP1 expression loss occurs in less than 20% of sarcomatoid mesothelioma.[64] Of note, in the absence of corroborative histologic features of malignancy (ie, invasion), aberrant BAP1 expression in mesothelial cells alone is not sufficient for the diagnosis of malignant mesothelioma. Mesothelioma in situ, as characterized by a single layer of surface mesothelial cells showing BAP1 expression loss with no evidence of invasion and absence of any pleural nodules or masses, has recently been described and may represent a precursor lesion to developing malignant mesothelioma, albeit with a protracted course in some cases.[74]

MTAP (methylthioadenosine phosphorylase) immunohistochemistry has been used as a diagnostic marker for malignant mesothelioma. MTAP is located near CDKN2A on the chromosomal region 9p21; loss of cytoplasmic MTAP staining is considered a surrogate for chromosomal 9p loss as determined by concurrent CDKN2A fluorescence in situ hybridization testing[75] and has been reported in approximately 40% to 60% of malignant mesothelioma but rarely in reactive proliferations.[61–63] In distinguishing malignant mesothelioma from reactive mesothelial proliferations, although MTAP alone is not sensitive, combined use of BAP1 and MTAP immunohistochemistry may improve the sensitivity and specificity.[61–63] Of note, because approximately 10% to 20% of lung adenocarcinoma shows MTAP loss,[62] MTAP immunohistochemistry is not specific in the distinction between malignant mesothelioma and lung carcinoma.

Additional markers, such as cyclin D1 and 5-hmC (5-hydroxymethylcytosine), have been explored as potential tools to distinguish malignant mesothelioma from reactive mesothelial proliferations, although their utility in clinical practice remains unclear. One study used tissue microarrays and found diffuse nuclear cyclin D1 staining, indicative of Hippo pathway activation, in most malignant mesotheliomas and minimal to focal cyclin D1 staining in reactive mesothelial proliferations.[76] Reduction of 5-hmC has been noted in diverse tumor types including malignant mesothelioma[77]; multifocal (>50%) loss of 5-hmC staining was seen in most malignant mesotheliomas but not reactive mesothelial proliferations in one study.[78]

ULTRASTRUCTURAL FEATURES

Electron microscopy is performed in fresh tumor tissue that is saved at the time of gross examination. In malignant mesothelioma, tumor cells characteristically display elongated microvilli, with a length-to-width ratio of greater than 10:1, on the luminal and abluminal surfaces.[79,80] Prominent desmosomes and abundant intermediate filaments are present. These ultrastructural features are prominent in epithelioid mesothelioma but is subtle to absent in sarcomatoid mesothelioma.[80]

CYTOGENETIC FEATURES

Most diffuse malignant pleural mesotheliomas are characterized by complex numerical and structural karyotypic alterations.[81] Although no specific chromosomal abnormalities are pathognomonic for malignant mesothelioma, loss of chromosomal region 9p including CDKN2A or 22q including NF2 is noted in a subset of tumors. With fluorescence in situ hybridization testing, homozygous loss of CDKN2A is found in approximately 60% of diffuse malignant pleural mesothelioma[82–84]; hemizygous loss of NF2 is present in approximately 50% of diffuse malignant pleural mesothelioma.[85] Although the presence of CDKN2A loss can aid the distinction of malignant mesothelioma from reactive mesothelial proliferations, CDKN2A loss alone is not useful in separating malignant mesothelioma from other tumor types, because CDKN2A loss is found in a substantial fraction of sarcomatoid mesothelioma, sarcomatoid carcinomas, and sarcomas.[86]

A rare subset of malignant pleural mesothelioma harbors a peculiar near-haploid karyotype, with extensive loss-of-heterozygosity involving nearly all chromosomes except chromosomes 5 and 7.[87]

MOLECULAR FEATURES

Most diffuse malignant pleural mesotheliomas are characterized by recurrent mutations in tumor suppressors and epigenetic regulators, including BAP1, NF2, TP53, SETD2, and others.[87–91] Alterations are identified in multiple pathways in the regulation of cell cycle, RNA processing, histone regulation, and cell growth.[89] BAP1 is one of the most frequently altered genes; mechanisms of BAP1 inactivation include point mutations, copy number loss, inactivating structural rearrangements, and minute chromosomal deletions.[87–89,92–94]

Furthermore, a small subset of diffuse malignant pleural mesothelioma harbors unusual genetic alterations: genomic near-haploidization has been described in rare malignant pleural mesotheliomas that harbor mutations in TP53 and/or SETDB1.[87] Oncogenic EWSR1-ATF1 fusion has been described in a malignant pleural mesothelioma from a young female.[95] Although ALK rearrangements have been identified in rare patients with diffuse malignant peritoneal mesothelioma,[96–98] this has not been identified in patients with diffuse malignant pleural mesothelioma.

Germline mutations are overall present in less than 10% of patients with diffuse malignant pleural mesothelioma and primarily involve genes in the DNA repair and cell cycle regulation, such as BAP1, BRCA2, CDKN2A, TMEM127, VHL, WT1, MRE11A, and MSH6.[99,100] Germline mutations seem to be enriched in patients who are young, with family history of mesothelioma, or with peritoneal mesothelioma.[99,101,102]

Consistent with its histomorphologic heterogeneity, diffuse malignant pleural mesothelioma shows an impressive molecular diversity. Several research groups have proposed various molecular classification schemes to establish molecular groups of malignant mesothelioma, using data from genomics, transcriptomics, proteomics, epigenomics, immune features, or a combination of these approaches.[87,89,103–105] In addition, one study analyzed the data using a decomposition approach and proposed a histo-molecular continuum in diffuse malignant pleural mesothelioma, with each tumor comprising epithelioid-like and sarcomatoid-like molecular features.[90]

DIFFERENTIAL DIAGNOSIS

The differential diagnosis of malignant pleural mesothelioma depends on the histologic type (epithelioid, biphasic, or sarcomatoid) under consideration (**Box 1**, **Figs. 4** and **5**). Diffuse malignant pleural mesothelioma can resemble reactive pleuritis or diverse tumor types, including carcinomas, melanoma, and sarcomas.

In addition to diffuse malignant pleural mesothelioma, the World Health Organization recognizes additional types of mesothelial lesions: localized malignant mesothelioma, well-differentiated papillary mesothelioma, and adenomatoid tumor.[1] Localized pleural mesothelioma is microscopically identical to diffuse malignant mesothelioma, although it is radiographically and grossly solitary and circumscribed[37–39]; genetically, localized pleural mesothelioma comprises three groups (BAP1-mutant, TRAF7-mutant, and near-haploid), with similarities but also differences from diffuse malignant pleural mesothelioma.[40] Well-differentiated papillary mesothelioma (see **Fig. 4**E), often an incidental finding in the peritoneum of women, can occur in the pleura[106] and is genetically characterized by recurrent mutations in TRAF7 or CDC42.[107] Rarely, well-differentiated papillary mesothelioma shows back-to-back papillae with foci of invasion,[108] morphologically mimicking diffuse malignant mesothelioma. Furthermore, distinction between a malignant mesothelioma with prominent papillary surface projections and well-differentiated papillary

Box 1
Differential diagnosis

Differential diagnosis of epithelioid malignant mesothelioma

- Metastatic carcinoma
  - Expresses epithelial markers (eg, claudin-4, MOC31, and MUC4)
  - Rarely or does not express mesothelial markers (eg, WT1, calretinin, and D2-40)
  - Most lung adenocarcinomas express TTF-1 and Napsin A
  - Most squamous cell carcinomas express p40 and p63
  - CK5/6 is expressed in squamous cell carcinoma and epithelioid mesothelioma and is not useful for distinction
  - Identification of genetic alterations characteristic of lung carcinomas (eg, EGFR activating or MET exon 14 skipping mutations) supports carcinomas and excludes sarcomatoid mesothelioma
- Metastatic melanoma
  - Variable architectural patterns and prominent nucleoli
  - Expresses melanocytic markers (eg, S-100 protein, SOX10, and HMB45)
- Epithelioid hemangioendothelioma
  - Rare distinctive malignant vascular tumor
  - Cord-like pattern, myxohyaline matrix, intracytoplasmic vacuoles
  - Expresses vascular markers (eg, ERG, CD31, and CD34) and CAMTA1 in most cases[134]
  - D2-40 is expressed in malignant mesothelioma and epithelioid hemangioendothelioma and is not useful for distinction
  - Recurrent WWTR1-CAMTA1 or rarely YAP1-TFE3 fusion[135,136]
- Well-differentiated papillary mesothelioma
  - Papillae with myxoid cores and single mesothelial cell layers
  - Recurrent TRAF7 or CDC42 mutations[107]
- Adenomatoid tumor
  - Microcystic architecture, with tubules and cords of epithelioid vacuolated cells
  - Recurrent TRAF7 mutations[109]

Differential diagnosis of sarcomatoid malignant mesothelioma

- Sarcomatoid carcinoma
  - Expresses epithelial markers (eg, claudin-4, MOC31, and MUC4)
  - Rarely or does not express mesothelial markers (eg, WT1, calretinin, and D2-40)
  - Aberrant BAP1 expression favors sarcomatoid mesothelioma over sarcomatoid carcinoma
  - Identification of genetic alterations characteristic of lung carcinomas (eg, EGFR activating or MET exon 14 skipping mutations) supports carcinomas and excludes sarcomatoid mesothelioma
- Chronic fibrosing pleuritis
  - Does not show dense cellularity, expansile nodules, or absence of zonation effect
  - Invasion is the most reliable criterion to exclude a reactive process and to confirm malignancy
- Synovial sarcoma
  - Monophasic, biphasic, or poorly differentiated histology
  - Recurrent SYT-SSX1 or SYT-SSX2 fusion in most cases[137]
  - TLE1 is expressed in synovial sarcoma and malignant mesothelioma[138] and is thus not specific for distinction
- Solitary fibrous tumor
  - Collagenous background, hemangiopericytoma-like staghorn vessels, and monomorphic spindle cells
  - Recurrent NAB2-STAT6 fusion[139,140]
  - Expresses STAT6 by immunohistochemistry[141]

Differential diagnosis of biphasic malignant mesothelioma

- Biphasic synovial sarcoma
  - Recurrent SYT-SSX1 fusion in most cases
  - TLE1 is expressed in synovial sarcoma and malignant mesothelioma[138] and is thus not specific for distinction
- Epithelioid hemangioendothelioma
  - Rare distinctive malignant vascular tumor
  - Cord-like pattern, myxohyaline matrix, intracytoplasmic vacuoles
  - Expresses vascular markers (eg, ERG, CD31, and CD34) and CAMTA1 in most cases[134]
  - D2-40 is expressed in malignant mesothelioma and epithelioid hemangioendothelioma and is not useful for distinction
  - Recurrent WWTR1-CAMTA1 or rarely YAP1-TFE3 fusion[135,136]

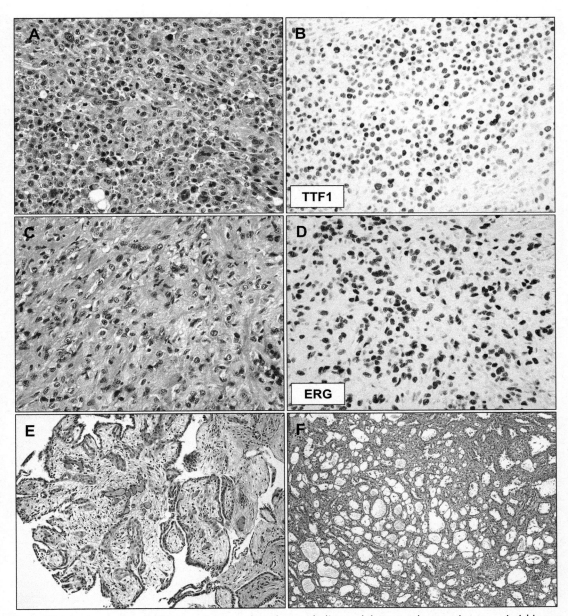

Fig. 4. Histologic mimics of diffuse malignant pleural mesothelioma. (*A*) Lung adenocarcinoma, mimicking an epithelioid mesothelioma. (*B*) Tumor cells in *A* show diffuse strong TTF1 expression and lacks mesothelial marker expression (not shown), confirming the diagnosis. (*C*) Epithelioid hemangioendothelioma, with cord-like growth pattern and rare vacuoles. (*D*) Tumor cells in *C* show diffuse strong ERG expression, along with expression of vascular markers CD31 and CAMTA1 (not shown), confirming the diagnosis. (*E*) Well-differentiated papillary mesothelioma, characterized by papillary architecture with each core lined by a single cell layer. (*F*) Adenomatoid tumor, characterized by a microcystic appearance with epithelioid-to-vacuolated tumor cells.

mesothelioma is challenging, particularly in small superficial biopsies. Adenomatoid tumor (see **Fig. 4**F) primarily affects the genital tracts but rarely can involve the pleura; recurrent mutations in *TRAF7* have been described in adenomatoid tumors of genital-type.[109]

EMERGING PROGNOSTIC AND PREDICTIVE FACTORS

In diffuse malignant pleural mesothelioma, histologic type is an integral prognostic indicator: patients with epithelioid, biphasic, and sarcomatoid

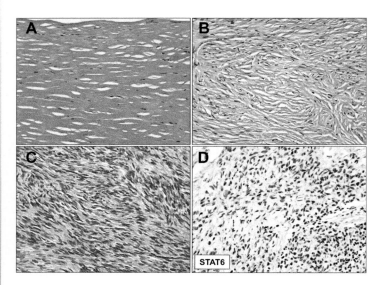

Fig. 5. Histologic mimics of diffuse malignant pleural mesothelioma. (*A*) Pleural plaque, showing orderly arrangement of mesothelial cells. (*B*) Desmoplastic mesothelioma, characterized by storiform arrangement of tumor cells, mimicking a pleural plaque or fibrosis. (*C*) Solitary fibrous tumor, mimicking sarcomatoid mesothelioma. (*D*) Tumor cells in *C* show diffuse strong STAT6 expression, along with absence of mesothelial marker expression (not shown), confirming the diagnosis.

mesotheliomas have an overall median survival of approximately 14, 10, and 5 months, respectively.[6,110,111] Over the years, additional histologic, immunohistochemical, molecular, and immune features have been described to be prognostic or predictive of select therapy.

In epithelioid mesothelioma, poor prognostic features described include the presence of micropapillary or solid patterns.[112] Pleomorphic mesothelioma is characterized by anaplasia and/or multinucleated tumor giant cells comprising at least 10% of the tumor.[113] Historically considered as a subtype of epithelioid mesothelioma including in the World Health Organization 2015 classification,[1] pleomorphic mesothelioma has an aggressive clinical behavior comparable with sarcomatoid mesothelioma.[114] Another emerging pattern to recognize is the transitional subtype, characterized by sheet-like growth of elongated plump tumor cells with well-defined cell borders and cohesion.[33] Although the histologic interobserver concordance is fair-to-moderate, transitional mesothelioma shows a poor prognosis comparable with sarcomatoid mesothelioma.[33,115] In addition to the assessment of architectural patterns, various three- or two-tiered grading schemes have been described over the years and include the assessment of mitotic activity, necrosis,[112,116–121] and, in one system, Ki67 proliferation index.[120] The recent European Reference Network for Rare Adult Solid Cancers/International Association for the Study of Lung Cancer proposal for histologic classification for epithelioid pleural mesothelioma has proposed that diagnostic reports should include the assessment of nuclear atypia, mitotic count, and necrosis and assign tumors into low and high grades.[122]

Recent studies explored immunohistochemical targets as potential prognostic and predictive markers. In a study of diffuse malignant pleural mesothelioma patients with epithelioid histology, prolonged survival has been noted in tumors with loss of BAP1 and retained p16 expression in univariate and multivariate analyses.[123] Certain molecular features seem to be prognostic in diffuse malignant pleural mesothelioma. In particular, patients with mesothelioma with germline *BAP1* mutations show a prolonged survival.[102,124] Patients with mesothelioma with germline mutations in one of the DNA repair genes also respond better to platinum chemotherapy as compared with patients without germline mutations,[100] thus highlighting the prognostic and predictive value of these mutations in patients with diffuse malignant pleural mesothelioma. Of note, although the presence of *ALK* gene rearrangements in rare patients with diffuse malignant peritoneal mesothelioma[96–98] raises the possibility of targeted treatment with ALK inhibitors,[125] this has not been demonstrated in patients with diffuse malignant pleural mesothelioma to date.

Programmed death-ligand 1 (PD-L1; CD274), a negative regulator of immune checkpoint, represents a target in immunotherapy, with PD-L1 immunohistochemistry evaluated as a predictive biomarker in diverse tumor types.[126] PD-L1 expression generally seems higher in sarcomatoid mesothelioma than in epithelioid mesothelioma.[127–130] Increased PD-L1 expression has been noted in sarcomatoid mesothelioma but not in reactive mesothelial proliferations,[131] suggesting PD-L1 immunohistochemistry as a potential tool to separate sarcomatoid mesothelioma from reactive mesothelial proliferations.[131] In terms of its predictive value, the utility of PD-L1 immunohistochemistry and optimal assessment criteria in diffuse malignant pleural mesothelioma remain unclear.

Epithelioid mesothelioma rarely expresses PD-L1 but seems to rely on VISTA (V-domain Ig Suppressor of T-cell Activation; VSIR [V-set immunoregulatory receptor]) for immune blockade.[87,90] Immunohistochemistry for VISTA shows high expression in epithelioid mesothelioma but not in sarcomatoid mesothelioma.[132,133] Because VISTA is expressed in benign mesothelial cells, VISTA immunohistochemistry cannot distinguish between malignant epithelioid mesothelioma and reactive mesothelial proliferations.[132] However, non–small cell lung carcinomas do not seem to express VISTA,[132] suggesting a potential diagnostic role of using VISTA immunohistochemistry to distinguish epithelioid mesothelioma from lung carcinomas. In patients with diffuse malignant pleural mesothelioma, whereas PD-L1 expression correlates with worse survival,[133] VISTA expression correlates with better survival[132,133] and may suggest potential immunotherapy targets in these patients.

CLINICS CARE POINTS

- Histologic diagnosis of malignant mesothelioma is based on assessment of architectural features.
- Histologic typing of malignant mesothelioma (into epithelioid, biphasic, and sarcomatoid types) is based on assessment of cytologic features and has prognostic value.
- A panel of immunohistochemical markers is needed to distinguish sarcomatoid mesothelioma from sarcomatoid carcinoma and mimics.
- Loss of nuclear BAP1 staining by immunohistochemistry is specific but not sensitive in distinguishing malignant mesothelioma from reactive mesothelial proliferations.
- Correlation with clinical, radiologic, and molecular features is helpful in certain challenging diagnostic situations.

DISCLOSURE

L.R. Chirieac undertakes medicolegal work related to mesothelioma. Y.P. Hung has nothing to disclose.

REFERENCES

1. Travis WD, Brambilla E, Burke A, et al. Pathology and genetics of tumors of the lung, pleura, thymus, and heart. 4th edition. Lyon (France): IARC Press; 2015.
2. Moolgavkar SH, Meza R, Turim J. Pleural and peritoneal mesotheliomas in SEER: age effects and temporal trends, 1973-2005. Cancer Causes Control 2009;20(6):935–44.
3. Beebe-Dimmer JL, Fryzek JP, Yee CL, et al. Mesothelioma in the United States: a Surveillance, Epidemiology, and End Results (SEER)-Medicare investigation of treatment patterns and overall survival. Clin Epidemiol 2016;8:743–50.
4. Delgermaa V, Takahashi K, Park EK, et al. Global mesothelioma deaths reported to the World Health Organization between 1994 and 2008. Bull World Health Organ 2011;89(10):716–24.
5. Mazurek JM, Syamlal G, Wood JM, et al. Malignant mesothelioma mortality—United States, 1999-2015. MMWR Morb Mortal Wkly Rep 2017;66(8):214–8.
6. Nelson DB, Rice DC, Niu J, et al. Long-term survival outcomes of cancer-directed surgery for malignant pleural mesothelioma: propensity score matching analysis. J Clin Oncol 2017;35(29):3354–62.
7. Vivero M, Bueno R, Chirieac LR. Clinicopathologic and genetic characteristics of young patients with pleural diffuse malignant mesothelioma. Mod Pathol 2018;31(1):122–31.
8. Robinson BW, Lake RA. Advances in malignant mesothelioma. N Engl J Med 2005;353(15):1591–603.
9. Friedberg JS, Culligan MJ, Tsao AS, et al. A proposed system toward standardizing surgical-based treatments for malignant pleural mesothelioma, from the Joint National Cancer Institute-International Association for the Study of Lung Cancer-Mesothelioma Applied Research Foundation Taskforce. J Thorac Oncol 2019;14(8):1343–53.
10. Gomez DR, Rimner A, Simone CB 2nd, et al. The use of radiation therapy for the treatment of malignant pleural mesothelioma: expert opinion from the National Cancer Institute Thoracic Malignancy Steering Committee, International Association for the Study of Lung Cancer, and Mesothelioma Applied Research Foundation. J Thorac Oncol 2019;14(7):1172–83.
11. Scherpereel A, Mazieres J, Greillier L, et al. Nivolumab or nivolumab plus ipilimumab in patients with relapsed malignant pleural mesothelioma (IFCT-1501 MAPS2): a multicentre, open-label, randomised, non-comparative, phase 2 trial. Lancet Oncol 2019;20(2):239–53.

12. Roushdy-Hammady I, Siegel J, Emri S, et al. Genetic-susceptibility factor and malignant mesothelioma in the Cappadocian region of Turkey. Lancet 2001;357(9254):444–5.

13. Cavazza A, Travis LB, Travis WD, et al. Post-irradiation malignant mesothelioma. Cancer 1996;77(7): 1379–85.

14. Chirieac LR, Barletta JA, Yeap BY, et al. Clinicopathologic characteristics of malignant mesotheliomas arising in patients with a history of radiation for Hodgkin and non-Hodgkin lymphoma. J Clin Oncol 2013;31(36):4544–9.

15. Hillerdal G, Berg J. Malignant mesothelioma secondary to chronic inflammation and old scars. Two new cases and review of the literature. Cancer 1985;55(9):1968–72.

16. Kodama Y, Hoshi S, Minami M, et al. Malignant mesothelioma associated with chronic empyema with elevation of serum CYFRA19: A case report. Biosci Trends 2008;2(6):250–4.

17. Attanoos RL, Churg A, Galateau-Salle F, et al. Malignant mesothelioma and its non-asbestos causes. Arch Pathol Lab Med 2018;142(6): 753–60.

18. Testa JR, Cheung M, Pei J, et al. Germline BAP1 mutations predispose to malignant mesothelioma. Nat Genet 2011;43(10):1022–5.

19. Xu J, Kadariya Y, Cheung M, et al. Germline mutation of Bap1 accelerates development of asbestos-induced malignant mesothelioma. Cancer Res 2014;74(16):4388–97.

20. Guo Z, Carbone M, Zhang X, et al. Improving the accuracy of mesothelioma diagnosis in China. J Thorac Oncol 2017;12(4):714–23.

21. Larsen BT, Klein JR, Hornychova H, et al. Diffuse intrapulmonary malignant mesothelioma masquerading as interstitial lung disease: a distinctive variant of mesothelioma. Am J Surg Pathol 2013;37(10):1555–64.

22. Husain AN, Colby T, Ordonez N, et al. Guidelines for pathologic diagnosis of malignant mesothelioma: 2012 update of the consensus statement from the International Mesothelioma Interest Group. Arch Pathol Lab Med 2013;137(5): 647–67.

23. Ordonez NG. Mesothelioma with rhabdoid features: an ultrastructural and immunohistochemical study of 10 cases. Mod Pathol 2006;19(3):373–83.

24. Ordonez NG. Deciduoid mesothelioma: report of 21 cases with review of the literature. Mod Pathol 2012;25(11):1481–95.

25. Ordonez NG. Mesotheliomas with small cell features: report of eight cases. Mod Pathol 2012; 25(5):689–98.

26. Wilson GE, Hasleton PS, Chatterjee AK. Desmoplastic malignant mesothelioma: a review of 17 cases. J Clin Pathol 1992;45(4):295–8.

27. Klebe S, Brownlee NA, Mahar A, et al. Sarcomatoid mesothelioma: a clinical-pathologic correlation of 326 cases. Mod Pathol 2010;23(3):470–9.

28. Henderson DW, Attwood HD, Constance TJ, et al. Lymphohistiocytoid mesothelioma: a rare lymphomatoid variant of predominantly sarcomatoid mesothelioma. Ultrastruct Pathol 1988;12(4): 367–84.

29. Yao DX, Shia J, Erlandson RA, et al. Lymphohistiocytoid mesothelioma: a clinical, immunohistochemical and ultrastructural study of four cases and literature review. Ultrastruct Pathol 2004;28(4): 213–28.

30. Galateau-Salle F, Attanoos R, Gibbs AR, et al. Lymphohistiocytoid variant of malignant mesothelioma of the pleura: a series of 22 cases. Am J Surg Pathol 2007;31(5):711–6.

31. Galateau Salle F, Le Stang N, Nicholson AG, et al. New insights on diagnostic reproducibility of biphasic mesotheliomas: a multi-institutional evaluation by the International Mesothelioma Panel From the MESOPATH Reference Center. J Thorac Oncol 2018;13(8):1189–203.

32. Brcic L, Vlacic G, Quehenberger F, et al. Reproducibility of malignant pleural mesothelioma histopathologic subtyping. Arch Pathol Lab Med 2018; 142(6):747–52.

33. Dacic S, Le Stang N, Husain A, et al. Interobserver variation in the assessment of the sarcomatoid and transitional components in biphasic mesotheliomas. Mod Pathol 2020;33(2):255–62.

34. Arrossi AV, Lin E, Rice D, et al. Histologic assessment and prognostic factors of malignant pleural mesothelioma treated with extrapleural pneumonectomy. Am J Clin Pathol 2008;130(5): 754–64.

35. Kao SC, Yan TD, Lee K, et al. Accuracy of diagnostic biopsy for the histological subtype of malignant pleural mesothelioma. J Thorac Oncol 2011; 6(3):602–5.

36. Chirieac LR, Hung YP, Foo WC, et al. Diagnostic value of biopsy sampling in predicting histology in patients with diffuse malignant pleural mesothelioma. Cancer 2019;125(23):4164–71.

37. Okike N, Bernatz PE, Woolner LB. Localized mesothelioma of the pleura: benign and malignant variants. J Thorac Cardiovasc Surg 1978;75(3): 363–72.

38. Allen TC, Cagle PT, Churg AM, et al. Localized malignant mesothelioma. Am J Surg Pathol 2005; 29(7):866–73.

39. Marchevsky AM, Khoor A, Walts AE, et al. Localized malignant mesothelioma, an unusual and poorly characterized neoplasm of serosal origin: best current evidence from the literature and the International Mesothelioma Panel. Mod Pathol 2020; 33(2):281–96.

40. Hung YP, Dong F, Dubuc AM, et al. Molecular characterization of localized pleural mesothelioma. Mod Pathol 2020;33(2):271–80.

41. Churg A, Colby TV, Cagle P, et al. The separation of benign and malignant mesothelial proliferations. Am J Surg Pathol 2000;24(9):1183–200.

42. Churg A, Galateau-Salle F. The separation of benign and malignant mesothelial proliferations. Arch Pathol Lab Med 2012;136(10):1217–26.

43. Churg A, Cagle P, Colby TV, et al. The fake fat phenomenon in organizing pleuritis: a source of confusion with desmoplastic malignant mesotheliomas. Am J Surg Pathol 2011;35(12):1823–9.

44. Ordonez NG. Immunohistochemical diagnosis of epithelioid mesothelioma: an update. Arch Pathol Lab Med 2005;129(11):1407–14.

45. Facchetti F, Gentili F, Lonardi S, et al. Claudin-4 in mesothelioma diagnosis. Histopathology 2007; 51(2):261–3.

46. Anttila S. Epithelioid lesions of the serosa. Arch Pathol Lab Med 2012;136(3):241–52.

47. Amatya VJ, Kushitani K, Kai Y, et al. Glypican-1 immunohistochemistry is a novel marker to differentiate epithelioid mesothelioma from lung adenocarcinoma. Mod Pathol 2018;31(5):809–15.

48. Tsuji S, Washimi K, Kageyama T, et al. HEG1 is a novel mucin-like membrane protein that serves as a diagnostic and therapeutic target for malignant mesothelioma. Sci Rep 2017;7:45768.

49. Naso JR, Tsuji S, Churg A. HEG1 is a highly specific and sensitive marker of epithelioid malignant mesothelioma. Am J Surg Pathol 2020. https://doi.org/10.1097/PAS.0000000000001469.

50. Amatya VJ, Kushitani K, Mawas AS, et al. MUC4, a novel immunohistochemical marker identified by gene expression profiling, differentiates pleural sarcomatoid mesothelioma from lung sarcomatoid carcinoma. Mod Pathol 2017;30(5):672–81.

51. Mawas AS, Amatya VJ, Kushitani K, et al. MUC4 immunohistochemistry is useful in distinguishing epithelioid mesothelioma from adenocarcinoma and squamous cell carcinoma of the lung. Sci Rep 2018;8(1):134.

52. Husain AN, Colby TV, Ordonez NG, et al. Guidelines for pathologic diagnosis of malignant mesothelioma 2017 Update of the Consensus Statement From the International Mesothelioma Interest Group. Arch Pathol Lab Med 2018;142(1):89–108.

53. Chirieac LR, Pinkus GS, Pinkus JL, et al. The immunohistochemical characterization of sarcomatoid malignant mesothelioma of the pleura. Am J Cancer Res 2011;1(1):14–24.

54. Marchevsky AM, LeStang N, Hiroshima K, et al. The differential diagnosis between pleural sarcomatoid mesothelioma and spindle cell/pleomorphic (sarcomatoid) carcinomas of the lung: evidence-based guidelines from the International Mesothelioma Panel and the MESOPATH National Reference Center. Hum Pathol 2017;67:160–8.

55. Le Stang N, Burke L, Blaizot G, et al. Differential diagnosis of epithelioid malignant mesothelioma with lung and breast pleural metastasis: a systematic review compared with a standardized panel of antibodies—a new proposal that may influence pathologic practice. Arch Pathol Lab Med 2020; 144(4):446–56.

56. Carbone M, Yang H, Pass HI, et al. BAP1 and cancer. Nat Rev Cancer 2013;13(3):153–9.

57. Sheffield BS, Hwang HC, Lee AF, et al. BAP1 immunohistochemistry and p16 FISH to separate benign from malignant mesothelial proliferations. Am J Surg Pathol 2015;39(7):977–82.

58. Cigognetti M, Lonardi S, Fisogni S, et al. BAP1 (BRCA1-associated protein 1) is a highly specific marker for differentiating mesothelioma from reactive mesothelial proliferations. Mod Pathol 2015; 28(8):1043–57.

59. Andrici J, Jung J, Sheen A, et al. Loss of BAP1 expression is very rare in peritoneal and gynecologic serous adenocarcinomas and can be useful in the differential diagnosis with abdominal mesothelioma. Hum Pathol 2016;51:9–15.

60. Carbone M, Shimizu D, Napolitano A, et al. Positive nuclear BAP1 immunostaining helps differentiate non-small cell lung carcinomas from malignant mesothelioma. Oncotarget 2016;7(37): 59314–21.

61. Hida T, Hamasaki M, Matsumoto S, et al. Immunohistochemical detection of MTAP and BAP1 protein loss for mesothelioma diagnosis: comparison with 9p21 FISH and BAP1 immunohistochemistry. Lung Cancer 2017;104:98–105.

62. Berg KB, Dacic S, Miller C, et al. Utility of methylthioadenosine phosphorylase compared with BAP1 immunohistochemistry, and CDKN2A and NF2 fluorescence in situ hybridization in separating reactive mesothelial proliferations from epithelioid malignant mesotheliomas. Arch Pathol Lab Med 2018;142(12):1549–53.

63. Kinoshita Y, Hamasaki M, Yoshimura M, et al. A combination of MTAP and BAP1 immunohistochemistry is effective for distinguishing sarcomatoid mesothelioma from fibrous pleuritis. Lung Cancer 2018;125:198–204.

64. Hwang HC, Sheffield BS, Rodriguez S, et al. Utility of BAP1 immunohistochemistry and p16 (CDKN2A) FISH in the diagnosis of malignant mesothelioma in effusion cytology specimens. Am J Surg Pathol 2016;40(1):120–6.

65. Misumi K, Hayashi A, Shibahara J, et al. Intrahepatic cholangiocarcinoma frequently shows loss of BAP1 and PBRM1 expression, and demonstrates specific clinicopathologic and genetic

characteristics with BAP1 loss. Histopathology 2017;70(5):766–74.

66. Joseph RW, Kapur P, Serie DJ, et al. Loss of BAP1 protein expression is an independent marker of poor prognosis in patients with low-risk clear cell renal cell carcinoma. Cancer 2014;120(7): 1059–67.

67. Andrici J, Parkhill TR, Jung J, et al. Loss of expression of BAP1 is very rare in non-small cell lung carcinoma. Pathology 2016;48(4):336–40.

68. Owen D, Sheffield BS, Ionescu D, et al. Loss of BRCA1-associated protein 1 (BAP1) expression is rare in non-small cell lung cancer. Hum Pathol 2017;60:82–5.

69. Padgett DM, Cathro HP, Wick MR, et al. Podoplanin is a better immunohistochemical marker for sarcomatoid mesothelioma than calretinin. Am J Surg Pathol 2008;32(1):123–7.

70. Berg KB, Churg A. GATA3 immunohistochemistry for distinguishing sarcomatoid and desmoplastic mesothelioma from sarcomatoid carcinoma of the lung. Am J Surg Pathol 2017; 41(9):1221–5.

71. Miettinen M, McCue PA, Sarlomo-Rikala M, et al. GATA3: a multispecific but potentially useful marker in surgical pathology: a systematic analysis of 2500 epithelial and nonepithelial tumors. Am J Surg Pathol 2014;38(1):13–22.

72. Churg A, Sheffield BS, Galateau-Salle F. New markers for separating benign from malignant mesothelial proliferations: are we there yet? Arch Pathol Lab Med 2016;140(4):318–21.

73. Lee AF, Gown AM, Churg A. IMP3 and GLUT-1 immunohistochemistry for distinguishing benign from malignant mesothelial proliferations. Am J Surg Pathol 2013;37(3):421–6.

74. Churg A, Galateau-Salle F, Roden AC, et al. Malignant mesothelioma in situ: morphologic features and clinical outcome. Mod Pathol 2020;33(2): 297–302.

75. Chapel DB, Schulte JJ, Berg K, et al. MTAP immunohistochemistry is an accurate and reproducible surrogate for CDKN2A fluorescence in situ hybridization in diagnosis of malignant pleural mesothelioma. Mod Pathol 2020;33(2):245–54.

76. Pors J, Naso J, Berg K, et al. Cyclin D1 immunohistochemical staining to separate benign from malignant mesothelial proliferations. Mod Pathol 2020; 33(2):312–8.

77. Roulois D, Deshayes S, Guilly MN, et al. Characterization of preneoplastic and neoplastic rat mesothelial cell lines: the involvement of TETs, DNMTs, and 5-hydroxymethylcytosine. Oncotarget 2016; 7(23):34664–87.

78. Chapel DB, Husain AN, Krausz T. Immunohistochemical evaluation of nuclear 5-hydroxymethylcytosine (5-hmC) accurately distinguishes malignant

pleural mesothelioma from benign mesothelial proliferations. Mod Pathol 2019;32(3):376–86.

79. Warhol MJ, Hickey WF, Corson JM. Malignant mesothelioma: ultrastructural distinction from adenocarcinoma. Am J Surg Pathol 1982;6(4): 307–14.

80. Oury TD, Hammar SP, Roggli VL. Ultrastructural features of diffuse malignant mesotheliomas. Hum Pathol 1998;29(12):1382–92.

81. Sandberg AA, Bridge JA. Updates on the cytogenetics and molecular genetics of bone and soft tissue tumors. Mesothelioma. Cancer Genet Cytogenet 2001;127(2):93–110.

82. Illei PB, Rusch VW, Zakowski MF, et al. Homozygous deletion of CDKN2A and codeletion of the methylthioadenosine phosphorylase gene in the majority of pleural mesotheliomas. Clin Cancer Res 2003;9(6):2108–13.

83. Dacic S, Kothmaier H, Land S, et al. Prognostic significance of p16/cdkn2a loss in pleural malignant mesotheliomas. Virchows Arch 2008;453(6): 627–35.

84. Chiosea S, Krasinskas A, Cagle PT, et al. Diagnostic importance of 9p21 homozygous deletion in malignant mesotheliomas. Mod Pathol 2008; 21(6):742–7.

85. Kinoshita Y, Hamasaki M, Yoshimura M, et al. Hemizygous loss of NF2 detected by fluorescence in situ hybridization is useful for the diagnosis of malignant pleural mesothelioma. Mod Pathol 2020; 33(2):235–44.

86. Tochigi N, Attanoos R, Chirieac LR, et al. p16 Deletion in sarcomatoid tumors of the lung and pleura. Arch Pathol Lab Med 2013;137(5):632–6.

87. Hmeljak J, Sanchez-Vega F, Hoadley KA, et al. Integrative molecular characterization of malignant pleural mesothelioma. Cancer Discov 2018;8(12): 1548–65.

88. Guo G, Chmielecki J, Goparaju C, et al. Whole-exome sequencing reveals frequent genetic alterations in BAP1, NF2, CDKN2A, and CUL1 in malignant pleural mesothelioma. Cancer Res 2015; 75(2):264–9.

89. Bueno R, Stawiski EW, Goldstein LD, et al. Comprehensive genomic analysis of malignant pleural mesothelioma identifies recurrent mutations, gene fusions and splicing alterations. Nat Genet 2016;48(4):407–16.

90. Blum Y, Meiller C, Quetel L, et al. Dissecting heterogeneity in malignant pleural mesothelioma through histo-molecular gradients for clinical applications. Nat Commun 2019;10(1):1333.

91. Quetel L, Meiller C, Assie JB, et al. Genetic alterations of malignant pleural mesothelioma: association to tumor heterogeneity and overall survival. Mol Oncol 2020. https://doi.org/10.1002/1878-0261. 12651.

92. Bott M, Brevet M, Taylor BS, et al. The nuclear deubiquitinase BAP1 is commonly inactivated by somatic mutations and 3p21.1 losses in malignant pleural mesothelioma. Nat Genet 2011;43(7): 668–72.

93. Lo Iacono M, Monica V, Righi L, et al. Targeted next-generation sequencing of cancer genes in advanced stage malignant pleural mesothelioma: a retrospective study. J Thorac Oncol 2015;10(3): 492–9.

94. Yoshikawa Y, Emi M, Hashimoto-Tamaoki T, et al. High-density array-CGH with targeted NGS unmask multiple noncontiguous minute deletions on chromosome 3p21 in mesothelioma. Proc Natl Acad Sci U S A 2016;113(47):13432–7.

95. Desmeules P, Joubert P, Zhang L, et al. A subset of malignant mesotheliomas in young adults are associated with recurrent EWSR1/FUS-ATF1 fusions. Am J Surg Pathol 2017;41(7):980–8.

96. Hung YP, Dong F, Watkins JC, et al. Identification of ALK rearrangements in malignant peritoneal mesothelioma. JAMA Oncol 2018;4(2):235–8.

97. Loharamtaweethong K, Puripat N, Aoonjai N, et al. Anaplastic lymphoma kinase (ALK) translocation in paediatric malignant peritoneal mesothelioma: a case report of novel ALK-related tumour spectrum. Histopathology 2016;68(4):603–7.

98. Mian I, Abdullaev Z, Morrow B, et al. Anaplastic lymphoma kinase gene rearrangement in children and young adults with mesothelioma. J Thorac Oncol 2020;15(3):457–61.

99. Panou V, Gadiraju M, Wolin A, et al. Frequency of germline mutations in cancer susceptibility genes in malignant mesothelioma. J Clin Oncol 2018; 36(28):2863–71.

100. Hassan R, Morrow B, Thomas A, et al. Inherited predisposition to malignant mesothelioma and overall survival following platinum chemotherapy. Proc Natl Acad Sci U S A 2019;116(18):9008–13.

101. Ohar JA, Cheung M, Talarchek J, et al. Germline BAP1 mutational landscape of asbestos-exposed malignant mesothelioma patients with family history of cancer. Cancer Res 2016;76(2):206–15.

102. Pastorino S, Yoshikawa Y, Pass HI, et al. A subset of mesotheliomas with improved survival occurring in carriers of BAP1 and other germline mutations. J Clin Oncol 2018;36. JCO2018790352.

103. de Reynies A, Jaurand MC, Renier A, et al. Molecular classification of malignant pleural mesothelioma: identification of a poor prognosis subgroup linked to the epithelial-to-mesenchymal transition. Clin Cancer Res 2014;20(5):1323–34.

104. Gordon GJ, Rockwell GN, Jensen RV, et al. Identification of novel candidate oncogenes and tumor suppressors in malignant pleural mesothelioma using large-scale transcriptional profiling. Am J Pathol 2005;166(6):1827–40.

105. Lopez-Rios F, Chuai S, Flores R, et al. Global gene expression profiling of pleural mesotheliomas: overexpression of aurora kinases and P16/CDKN2A deletion as prognostic factors and critical evaluation of microarray-based prognostic prediction. Cancer Res 2006;66(6):2970–9.

106. Galateau-Salle F, Vignaud JM, Burke L, et al. Well-differentiated papillary mesothelioma of the pleura: a series of 24 cases. Am J Surg Pathol 2004;28(4): 534–40.

107. Stevers M, Rabban JT, Garg K, et al. Well-differentiated papillary mesothelioma of the peritoneum is genetically defined by mutually exclusive mutations in TRAF7 and CDC42. Mod Pathol 2019; 32(1):88–99.

108. Churg A, Allen T, Borczuk AC, et al. Well-differentiated papillary mesothelioma with invasive foci. Am J Surg Pathol 2014;38(7):990–8.

109. Goode B, Joseph NM, Stevers M, et al. Adenomatoid tumors of the male and female genital tract are defined by TRAF7 mutations that drive aberrant NF-kB pathway activation. Mod Pathol 2018;31(4): 660–73.

110. Sugarbaker DJ, Flores RM, Jaklitsch MT, et al. Resection margins, extrapleural nodal status, and cell type determine postoperative long-term survival in trimodality therapy of malignant pleural mesothelioma: results in 183 patients. J Thorac Cardiovasc Surg 1999;117(1):54–63 [discussion: 63–5].

111. Verma V, Ahern CA, Berlind CG, et al. Survival by histologic subtype of malignant pleural mesothelioma and the impact of surgical resection on overall survival. Clin Lung Cancer 2018;19(6):e901–12.

112. Rosen LE, Karrison T, Ananthanarayanan V, et al. Nuclear grade and necrosis predict prognosis in malignant epithelioid pleural mesothelioma: a multi-institutional study. Mod Pathol 2018;31(4): 598–606.

113. Ordonez NG. Pleomorphic mesothelioma: report of 10 cases. Mod Pathol 2012;25(7):1011–22.

114. Kadota K, Suzuki K, Sima CS, et al. Pleomorphic epithelioid diffuse malignant pleural mesothelioma: a clinicopathological review and conceptual proposal to reclassify as biphasic or sarcomatoid mesothelioma. J Thorac Oncol 2011;6(5):896–904.

115. Salle FG, Le Stang N, Tirode F, et al. Comprehensive molecular and pathological evaluation of transitional mesothelioma assisted by deep learning approach: a multi institutional study of the International Mesothelioma Panel from MESOPATH Reference Center. J Thorac Oncol 2020. https://doi.org/10.1016/j.jtho.2020.01.025.

116. Beer TW, Carr NJ, Whittaker MA, et al. Mitotic and in situ end-labeling apoptotic indices as prognostic markers in malignant mesothelioma. Ann Diagn Pathol 2000;4(3):143–8.

117. Borczuk AC, Taub RN, Hesdorffer M, et al. P16 loss and mitotic activity predict poor survival in patients with peritoneal malignant mesothelioma. Clin Cancer Res 2005;11(9):3303–8.

118. Demirag F, Unsal E, Yilmaz A, et al. Prognostic significance of vascular endothelial growth factor, tumor necrosis, and mitotic activity index in malignant pleural mesothelioma. Chest 2005;128(5):3382–7.

119. Kadota K, Suzuki K, Colovos C, et al. A nuclear grading system is a strong predictor of survival in epitheloid diffuse malignant pleural mesothelioma. Mod Pathol 2012;25(2):260–71.

120. Pelosi G, Papotti M, Righi L, et al. Pathologic grading of malignant pleural mesothelioma: an evidence-based proposal. J Thorac Oncol 2018;13(11):1750–61.

121. Zhang YZ, Brambilla C, Molyneaux PL, et al. Utility of nuclear grading system in epithelioid malignant pleural mesothelioma in biopsy-heavy setting: an external validation study of 563 cases. Am J Surg Pathol 2020;44(3):347–56.

122. Nicholson AG, Sauter JL, Nowak AK, et al. EURACAN/IASLC proposals for updating the histologic classification of pleural mesothelioma: towards a more multidisciplinary approach. J Thorac Oncol 2020;15(1):29–49.

123. Chou A, Toon CW, Clarkson A, et al. The epithelioid BAP1-negative and p16-positive phenotype predicts prolonged survival in pleural mesothelioma. Histopathology 2018;72(3):509–15.

124. Baumann F, Flores E, Napolitano A, et al. Mesothelioma patients with germline BAP1 mutations have 7-fold improved long-term survival. Carcinogenesis 2015;36(1):76–81.

125. Ruschoff JH, Gradhand E, Kahraman A, et al. STRN-ALK rearranged malignant peritoneal mesothelioma with dramatic response following ceritinib treatment. JCO Precis Oncol 2019;3:1–6.

126. Postow MA, Callahan MK, Wolchok JD. Immune checkpoint blockade in cancer therapy. J Clin Oncol 2015;33(17):1974–82.

127. Mansfield AS, Roden AC, Peikert T, et al. B7-H1 expression in malignant pleural mesothelioma is associated with sarcomatoid histology and poor prognosis. J Thorac Oncol 2014;9(7):1036–40.

128. Cedres S, Ponce-Aix S, Zugazagoitia J, et al. Analysis of expression of programmed cell death 1 ligand 1 (PD-L1) in malignant pleural mesothelioma (MPM). PLoS One 2015;10(3):e0121071.

129. Combaz-Lair C, Galateau-Salle F, McLeer-Florin A, et al. Immune biomarkers PD-1/PD-L1 and TLR3 in malignant pleural mesotheliomas. Hum Pathol 2016;52:9–18.

130. Thapa B, Salcedo A, Lin X, et al. The immune microenvironment, genome-wide copy number aberrations, and survival in mesothelioma. J Thorac Oncol 2017;12(5):850–9.

131. Derakhshan F, Ionescu D, Cheung S, et al. Use of programmed death ligand-1 (PD-L1) staining to separate sarcomatoid malignant mesotheliomas from benign mesothelial reactions. Arch Pathol Lab Med 2020;144(2):185–8.

132. Chung YS, Kim M, Cha YJ, et al. Expression of V-set immunoregulatory receptor in malignant mesothelioma. Mod Pathol 2020;33(2):263–70.

133. Muller S, Victoria Lai W, Adusumilli PS, et al. V-domain Ig-containing suppressor of T-cell activation (VISTA), a potentially targetable immune checkpoint molecule, is highly expressed in epithelioid malignant pleural mesothelioma. Mod Pathol 2020;33(2):303–11.

134. Doyle LA, Fletcher CD, Hornick JL. Nuclear expression of CAMTA1 distinguishes epithelioid hemangioendothelioma from histologic mimics. Am J Surg Pathol 2016;40(1):94–102.

135. Antonescu CR, Le Loarer F, Mosquera JM, et al. Novel YAP1-TFE3 fusion defines a distinct subset of epithelioid hemangioendothelioma. Genes Chromosomes Cancer 2013;52(8):775–84.

136. Errani C, Zhang L, Sung YS, et al. A novel WWTR1-CAMTA1 gene fusion is a consistent abnormality in epithelioid hemangioendothelioma of different anatomic sites. Genes Chromosomes Cancer 2011;50(8):644–53.

137. Clark J, Rocques PJ, Crew AJ, et al. Identification of novel genes, SYT and SSX, involved in the t(X;18)(p11.2;q11.2) translocation found in human synovial sarcoma. Nat Genet 1994;7(4):502–8.

138. Matsuyama A, Hisaoka M, Iwasaki M, et al. TLE1 expression in malignant mesothelioma. Virchows Arch 2010;457(5):577–83.

139. Chmielecki J, Crago AM, Rosenberg M, et al. Whole-exome sequencing identifies a recurrent NAB2-STAT6 fusion in solitary fibrous tumors. Nat Genet 2013;45(2):131–2.

140. Robinson DR, Wu YM, Kalyana-Sundaram S, et al. Identification of recurrent NAB2-STAT6 gene fusions in solitary fibrous tumor by integrative sequencing. Nat Genet 2013;45(2):180–5.

141. Doyle LA, Vivero M, Fletcher CD, et al. Nuclear expression of STAT6 distinguishes solitary fibrous tumor from histologic mimics. Mod Pathol 2014;27(3):390–5.

The Molecular Basis of Malignant Pleural Mesothelioma

Benjamin Wadowski, MD, Assunta De Rienzo, PhD, Raphael Bueno, MD*

KEYWORDS

• Mesothelioma • Molecular • Genetic • Gene expression • Epigenetic

KEY POINTS

- Malignant pleural mesothelioma (MPM) is highly heterogeneous at the molecular level, leading to challenges in diagnosis, prognosis, and treatment.
- MPM is associated with asbestos exposure in greater than 80% of cases. Mechanisms of asbestos-associated tumorigenesis include reactive oxygen species, chronic inflammation, direct cytotoxicity, and cytokine and growth factor dysregulation.
- Epigenetic hallmarks of MPM include widespread chromosomal loss and aberrant gene methylation, although these patterns are complex and variable.
- MPM is characterized by the presence of fewer protein-altering somatic point-mutations compared with other cancers. Key mutated genes include tumor suppressors *BAP1*, *NF2*, *CDKN2A/B*, *TP53*, and *SETD2*.
- Integrated multi-omic analyses identify up to 4 distinct clusters of MPM, with 2 extreme epithelioid-like and mesenchymal-like groups separated by molecular gradient along the epithelial-to-mesenchymal transition spectrum.

INTRODUCTION

Malignant pleural mesothelioma (MPM) is a rare but aggressive cancer associated with asbestos exposure in greater than 80% of cases.[1] It is almost uniformly lethal, and although decreasing use of asbestos has led to a plateau of incidence in Western countries, a long latency period after exposure combined with continued global asbestos use makes MPM an ongoing area of concern.[2] MPM is classified into 3 histologic subtypes: epithelioid, sarcomatoid, and biphasic. Epithelioid histology confers the most favorable prognosis and sarcomatoid the least, and a greater proportion of epithelial differentiation in biphasic tumors correlates with longer survival.[3,4]

At the molecular level, MPM is a highly heterogeneous disease both between patients and within individual tumors.[5–8] Intratumor heterogeneity can be further conceptualized as a combination of longitudinal (change over time) and spatial (among samples of the same tumor) heterogeneity.[7] The broad molecular variation seen in MPM and its microenvironment poses a significant challenge in diagnosis, prognostication, and treatment of this devastating disease. Although advances in molecular oncology have led to effective novel therapeutics for several solid organ cancers, first-line medical therapy for MPM in the form of cytotoxic combination cisplatin/pemetrexed-based chemotherapy has remained unchanged for decades.[9,10] The application of surgery and hemithoracic radiation in multimodal approaches

Division of Thoracic Surgery, Brigham and Women's Hospital, Harvard Medical School, 75 Francis Street, Boston, MA 02115, USA
* Corresponding author.
E-mail address: rbueno@bwh.harvard.edu

Thorac Surg Clin 30 (2020) 383–393
https://doi.org/10.1016/j.thorsurg.2020.08.005
1547-4127/20/© 2020 Elsevier Inc. All rights reserved.

prolongs survival only in a subset of patients, and the ability to accurately predict patient response to any form of treatment is limited.[9,11]

Next-generation sequencing technology and novel computational techniques combined with international collaborative efforts have resulted in greater understanding of the molecular basis of MPM. This article describes current molecular mechanisms behind MPM tumorigenesis, reviews the epigenetic, genetic, and transcriptomic hallmarks of MPM, and discusses the implications of advances in MPM molecular biology in clinical practice.

CURRENT EVIDENCE AND RESEARCH
Tumorigenesis

MPM arises from malignant transformation of the mesothelial cell monolayer on the surface of the parietal pleura. Approximately 70% to 90% of cases are associated with exposure to asbestos fibers.[12,13] Most research into asbestos as a cause of MPM relies on self-report of exposure, and quantitative data on the relation of asbestos exposure to mesothelioma risk are rare.[14]

Asbestos, unlike chemical carcinogens, exerts its effects over a long period, which is consistent with the 10- to 40-year latency period between estimated exposure and MPM diagnosis.[15] There is debate over the specific mechanisms through which asbestos causes mesothelioma.[6] Implicated pathways include generation of reactive oxygen species (ROS), direct cytotoxicity, kinase-mediated signaling, chronic inflammation, and cytokine and growth factor dysregulation.[6,13,16] A small subset of MPM tumors exhibit a distinctive widespread loss of heterozygosity, which may be consistent with spindle damage induced directly by asbestos fibers as well.[2] It is also likely that these mechanisms overlap and that no single pathway can be identified as a sole sufficient cause of malignant transformation.

Reactive oxygen species
Asbestos fibers generate ROS both directly and indirectly (eg, through immune-mediated inflammation). These asbestos fibers in turn lead to epigenetic and somatic genetic changes in mesothelial cells.[17] At the epigenetic level, increased ROS causes altered DNA methylation.[17] In vitro treatment of Met5A cells with asbestos, for example, resulted in significant methylation changes in CpG islands located in the promoter regions of genes involved in migration/cell adhesion. However, no correlation between changes in methylation and expression of these genes was observed except for a significant inverse

correlation with *DKK1*, whose protein is an antagonist of the Wnt/β-catenin signaling pathway.[18] Interestingly, in the absence of asbestos, in vitro treatment of MPM cell lines with exemestane, an aromatase inhibitor that generates ROS, had an antiproliferative effect.[19]

Downstream effects of environmental stress: mutagenesis and failure of DNA repair
MPM has a relatively low rate of somatic mutation compared with other solid cancers.[5] However, whether through ROS or other molecular mechanisms, asbestos fibers are clearly mutagenic at the chromosomal and gene levels in both in vitro and in vivo models, leading to tumorigenesis.[16,20] These damage patterns are consistent with known frequent alterations in DNA repair genes.[5] In contrast, asbestos-induced pleural thickening and plaques are produced by changes in gene regulation secondary to inflammation and ROS without mutagenesis,[16,21,22] suggesting that mutagenesis is a key step in development of asbestos-induced MPM. However, whether there is a threshold of asbestos exposure below which cancer does not develop remains controversial and likely depends on patient-specific genetic factors.[16,23]

Although chronic inflammation is implicated in MPM development, the role of inflammation-related genes in development of MPM following asbestos exposure is still controversial. Crovella and colleagues[23] investigated the role of 93 genetic variants in 12 genes encoding inflammasome and iron metabolism proteins in relation to the number of asbestos bodies (ABs), considered a hallmark of asbestos exposure, in 81 patients who died of MPM. Although there was no association between the number of ABs and most of the selected genes, the frequency of the single nucleotide polymorphism rs12150220 A/T (17p13.2) in the NLRP1 gene correlated with a significantly lower number of ABs, suggesting that NLRP1 inflammasome may contribute in the development of lung ABs. A subsequent analysis by the same group found no association between polymorphisms in *NLRP1* or *NLRP3* and susceptibility to MPM in asbestos-exposed individuals.[24]

Nonasbestos causes of malignant pleural mesothelioma
Despite the myriad of pathways through which asbestos can cause MPM, the risk of developing MPM among high-risk individuals with industrial asbestos exposure is only ~5%.[25] Other factors have been associated with mesothelioma: nonasbestos mineral fibers (eg, erionite, fluoroedenite, carbon nanotubes), therapeutic radiation, chronic

pleural inflammation, and (in rare cases) germline genetic mutations.[12] Apart from germline mutations, a definitive molecular signature to differentiate these causes has not yet been developed.

Epigenetics

Chromosomal losses

Aneuploidy, particularly chromosomal loss, is an epigenetic hallmark of MPM.[7,26–28] However, the copy number alteration (CNA) profiles of individual tumors are complex.[29] In one analysis of CNAs in 53 primary MPM tumor samples, 77% demonstrated a predominance of losses and 23% a predominance of gains.[30] The most common losses are in 1p, 3p14-p21, whole chromosome 4, 6q, 9p, and 22q.[7,26,27] None of these losses individually predominate in MPM. The frequencies of common losses include 9p21 (34%), 22q (32%), 4q31-32 (29%), 4p12-13 (25%), and 3p21 (16%).[28] These regions contain some of the most commonly mutated genes in MPM, including BAP1 (3p), CDKN2A (9p), and NF2 (22q).[7]

In addition to large chromosomal losses, focal losses have been described. For example, in the Guo and colleagues[27] series, deletion of 9p21 containing CDKN2A/2B was identified. In The Cancer Genome Atlas (TCGA) analysis,[2] focal copy number deletions were found to affect canonical MPM tumor suppressor genes, including CDKN2A (>50% of samples) and NF2 (>70%). Deletions of CDKN2A often involve the adjacent gene MTAP, which has been linked to increased sensitivity to pharmacologic inhibition.[2] Loss of CDKN2A was also associated with shorter overall survival.[2]

The TCGA analysis also identified a rare MPM subtype in a small number of tumors exhibiting genomic near-haploidization, absent alteration in BAP1, PBRM1, or SETD2, and universal inactivation of SETDB1. Women were overrepresented in this subtype (4 Females:1 Male), whereas histologic subtype showed no difference from the MPM cohort at large.[2]

Chromosomal gains

Although less common than losses, gains in some MPM chromosomal regions have been described. In one comparative genomic hybridization (CGH) analysis of 26 MPM tumors, 7 (27%) were found to have recurrent gains in 17q, involving known cancer-related genes, such as MAP3K3, SMARCD2, ERN1, and PRKCA.[31] Krismann and colleagues[28] examined 90 MPM cases using CGH and DNA cytometry, finding common gains in 8q22-23 (18%), 1q23/1q32 (16%), 7p14-15 (14%), and 15q22-25 (14%). An analysis of 41 epithelioid MPM revealed relative gains in the regions encompassing KDM5A (12p13), DVL1 (1p36), and MYC (8q24) compared with peritoneal mesothelioma samples.[32]

Chromosomal alterations by histologic subtype

In the Krismann cohort,[28] aneuploidy was significantly less frequently in sarcomatoid samples (75%) and significantly more frequently in epithelioid samples (88%), although absolute differences were small. Imbalances were detected by CGH in 84% of all samples with an average of 6.2 defects per sample. Losses of chromosomal regions were twice as frequent as gains, consistent with observations in other studies.[30] Epithelioid MPM had distinct recurrent losses at several locations, including 3p21 (33% vs 16% in the whole cohort) and 17p12-pter (26%); sarcomatoid MPM had distinct recurrent losses at 7q31-qter (21%) and 15q (18%). Biphasic tumors demonstrated a CGH pattern consistent with a combination of the other 2 subtypes.[28]

Changes in gene regulation

Dysregulation of epigenetic control of tumor suppressor genes is also present in MPM, particularly hypermethylation.[33] In a high-throughput global screening analysis for aberrant DNA hypermethylation in 50 MPM specimens, an average of 6.3% of genes was found to be hypermethylated in MPM compared with 8.8% in lung adenocarcinoma.[34] Methylation patterns were distinct between the two tumors based on hierarchical cluster analysis, and three of the hypermethylated genes (TMEM30 B, KAZALD1, and MAPK13) were unique to MPM, suggesting a potential role for these genes as diagnostic markers.[34] Interestingly, four patients included in this study showed low levels of gene methylation and longer survival, suggesting that methylation may affect the progression of this disease. In addition, the number of methylated genes increased significantly in stages III and IV disease compared with stages I and II.[34] An analysis published in the same year by Christensen and colleagues[35] identified distinct epigenetic profiles between normal pleura and MPM. These data suggest a unique epigenetic landscape in MPM compared with other forms of thoracic disease.[33–35]

Several key genes mutated in MPM are involved in epigenetic regulation. For example, in the Bueno cohort,[5] 8% of tumors exhibited mutations in SETD2, which encodes a histone methyltransferase, often leading to loss of function. Mutations in the SETDB1 and SETD5 histone methyltransferase genes were also identified. The downstream effects of these and other mutations in genes involved in epigenetic programming have not yet been fully elucidated. However, for example, *ITGA7* is a known tumor suppressor gene that may be epigenetically regulated, and decreased expression of ITGA7 has been associated with decreased overall survival in MPM.[36] Tsou and colleagues[33] evaluated 52 MPM samples using the MethylLight technique for 28 methylation markers and found significant changes in methylation in the *ESR1* (increased) and *APC* (decreased) loci, which are known to be involved in tumorigenesis. Similarly, tumors without DNA losses affecting *DNMT1*, a methyltransferase, exhibited higher average methylation indicating a significant change in the epigenetic landscape.[37]

Small noncoding microRNAs (miRNAs) also participate in posttranscriptional regulation of gene expression; irreversible alterations in miRNA expression are associated with cancer development.[17] miR-126 in particular is known to play a crucial role in MPM pathogenesis, where it fails to act as an oncosuppressor by inhibition of the PI3K/AKT pathway. Treatment with exogenous miR-126 under these circumstances results in tumor suppression in vitro.[17] Over the last decade, the biological activity of many other miR-NAs has been associated with MPM, including in the roles of tumor suppressor (miR-16-5p and miR-193a-3p) and cellular function (miR-182-5p, miR-183-5p, miR-24-3p) (reviewed in Reid and colleagues,[38] 2020).

DNA Mutation Signatures

Somatic mutations

As previously described, MPM has a relatively low rate of protein-altering somatic point mutations compared with other solid cancers.[5] In a cohort of 74 MPM tumors, whole-exome sequencing confirmed an overall rate of less than two nonsynonymous mutations per megabase in all but one sample[2] and demonstrated that MPM had a lower rate of protein-altering mutations than many other cancers except thyroid carcinoma and acute myeloid leukemia.[5]

In the Bueno series, targeted (n = 103) and whole-exome (n = 99) sequencing of paired MPM tumors revealed an average of 24 ± 11 protein-coding alterations per sample with no significant differences between molecular subtypes.[5] Quetel and colleagues[39] demonstrated in 49 MPM primary cultures and in 35 frozen tumor specimens that mutations in MPM exhibit an enrichment in C > T transitions. A recent review summarizing massively parallel sequencing studies has observed that genetic variations tend to cluster in the TP53/DNA repair pathway and the PI3K/AKT pathway.[29] Recent high-throughput analyses have identified recurrent mutations in several genes, which underlie key features of MPM molecular biology.

Somatic mutations: BAP1 and other tumor suppressors

The main recurrent genetic alterations in MPM have been identified in tumor suppressor genes. The most frequently mutated gene in most series is *BRCA1-Associated Protein 1* (*BAP1*), which is located in 3p21 (a region frequently lost in MPM) and altered in up to 60% of tumors.[2,5,26,30,40,41] *BAP1* encodes a deubiquitinating enzyme involved in DNA repair, cell cycle, cellular differentiation, and DNA damage response.[42–44] BAP1 also promotes apoptosis in wild-type cells through deubiquitylation and stabilization of the IP3R3 channel.[45] Loss of nuclear BAP1 expression by immunohistochemistry (IHC) is currently used as a diagnostic marker in MPM. However, although loss of nuclear BAP1 staining can sometimes distinguish reactive versus neoplastic stroma particularly in biphasic tumors, BAP1 staining even within MPM is known to be heterogeneous.[46,47] There is also evidence that *BAP1*-mutant malignancies may be sensitive to epigenetically based therapies.[48] However, patient survival does not correlate with presence of *BAP1* mutation itself.[2] In addition, MPM patients with germline *BAP1* mutations have fewer chromosomal alterations than others.[2,49]

Beyond *BAP1*, frequently mutated tumor suppressor genes in MPM include *CDKN2A*, *CDKN2B*, *NF2*, and *TP53*.[2,5,26,50] Seven additional significantly mutated genes, *SETD2*, *ULK2*, *CFAP45*, *SETDB1*, *RYR2*, *DDX51*, and *DDX3X*, were identified in the Bueno cohort.[5] Mutations in *TP53* were absent in epithelioid tumors. In this cohort, patients carrying *TP53* mutation showed lower overall survival compared with patients with wild-type *TP53* (*P* = .0167). Another analysis of 49 MPM primary cell lines and 35 frozen tumors for 22 genes confirmed the high frequency of *BAP1*, *NF2*, *CDKN2A/B*, *TP53*, and *SETD2* mutations in MPM.[39]

Another gene frequently mutated in MPM is *LATS2*, a member of the *Hippo* signaling pathway.[39] An analysis found alteration in *LATS2* in 11% of 61 MPM primary cell lines.[51] Mutations in *NF2* gene, another member of the Hippo pathway, were found to co-occur with *LATS2* mutations in 8% of the cases. Although other studies did not report a high rate of *LATS2* mutation, large deletions of chromosome 13, where *LATS2* resides, may indicate potential loss of this gene and possible underestimation of the prevalence of *LATS* alterations.[51]

Germline mutations

Germline mutations have been identified in up to 7-12% of patients with MPM.[52–54] Pleural site in general is less frequently associated with germline mutations than other primary mesothelioma sites.[52] Few studies have shown that germline mutation frequency increases with decreasing age at diagnosis.[52,54] In addition, patients with germline mutations are less likely to report asbestos exposure, more likely to report a second cancer diagnosis, and more likely to have epithelioid histology.[52,54]

Pathogenic germline variants in MPM are often involved in DNA damage repair and chromatin remodeling pathways, and BAP1 is the most frequently identified germline mutation.[52,54,55] Germline mutations in BAP1 are known to predispose families to mesothelioma.[56] BAP1 is also known to be frequently inactivated in cancers, such as uveal melanoma, clear cell renal cancer, and cholangiocarcinoma.[57] Taken together, loss-of-function germline mutations in BAP1 constitute what is termed the familial BAP1 syndrome, including MPM, uveal melanoma, cutaneous melanoma, and other dermatologic tumors, as well as renal cell carcinoma and meningioma.[58,59] MPM patients with germline BAP1 mutations almost always exhibit a second somatic BAP1 mutation leading to likely complete loss of function.[53] Germline BAP1 mutation is associated with less aggressive disease than sporadic MPM.[60]

Hassan and colleagues[53] investigated the impact of inherited loss-of-function mutations on survival in mesothelioma following platinum-based chemotherapy. In a cohort of 385 MPM patients, they found significantly longer overall survival following platinum-based chemotherapy in patients with any germline mutation, including BAP1, compared with patients without germline mutations (7.9 years vs 2.4 years, $P = .0012$). The benefit was comparable across all the genes under investigation. Interestingly, the effect of genotype was significant for pleural, but not peritoneal mesothelioma. In addition, there was no difference in tumor histology or reported asbestos exposure between the germline mutant and control patients. Overall, these results suggest that MPM patients with germline mutations in DNA repair and other tumor suppressor genes may benefit from platinum chemotherapy.[53] There is also evidence that the presence of germline mutations may predict sensitivity to PARP inhibition.[53,61]

Application of gene mutations to diagnosis

MPM subtypes may be difficult to distinguish from benign pleural proliferation and from other tumors, such as adenocarcinoma (for epithelioid MPM) and sarcoma (for sarcomatoid MPM).[62] No single IHC stain is diagnostic, and agreement among expert pathologists classifying histologically biphasic MPM is moderate at best.[63] Homozygous deletion of CDKN2A by fluorescent in situ hybridization (FISH) can be useful in distinguishing benign florid stromal reaction from sarcomatoid components of biphasic MPM tumors.[64] Because chromosomal losses of CDKN2A often involve the adjacent gene MTAP, and IHC for MTAP correlates well with CDKN2A FISH, it has been suggested that IHC for MTAP may be clinically useful in diagnosis of MPM.[2,63]

Characterization of Gene Expression

Recent advances in gene expression profiling have allowed for the simultaneous analysis of thousands of genes. Gene expression data have been applied across major cancer types to identify novel subtypes, predict outcomes, and define heterogeneity and the need for personalized treatments.[65]

Some of the first molecular MPM classifications were generated in the early 2000s primarily using microarrays.[66–69] Microarray data have also been used to identify candidate tumor-associated genes. For example, an analysis of miRNA dysregulation implicated CDKN2A, NF2, JUN, HGF, and PDGF2A as frequently affected in mesothelioma.[70] A subsequent meta-analysis of several sets of microarray data defined a list of potential novel biomarkers for MPM, including PTGS2, BIRC5, ASS1, JUNB, MCM2, AURKA, FGF2, MKI67, CAV1, SFRP1, CCNB1, CDK4, and MSLN.[71]

Several efforts have been made over the years to classify MPM tumors according to molecular characteristics. Gordon and colleagues[72] used expression arrays to analyze 40 MPM tumors as well as normal pleura, normal lung, and MPM cell lines. Unsupervised hierarchical clustering revealed two distinct groups of tumor samples that correlated loosely with tumor histology. Suraokar and colleagues[73] used microarray and pathway analysis to define three molecular subgroups of MPM, which correlated only partially with histologic subtypes.

Another analysis was published by de Reynies and colleagues[74] in 2014. This group investigated microarray profiles of 67 MPM cell lines and generated 2 MPM subclasses (termed C1 and C2) partially related to histologic type and closely related to prognosis. These clusters were characterized by the differential expression of epithelial-to-mesenchymal (EMT) genes with C1 expressing an epithelial and C2 a mesenchymal phenotype. C1 was characterized by more frequent *BAP1* and *CDKN2A* mutations, whereas C2 contained all the sarcomatoid/desmoplastic samples among other subtypes of MPM. The investigators created a predictor tool to discriminate samples between C1 and C2 using the expression levels of three genes: *PPL*, *UPK3B*, and *TFPI*. This tool was then used to validate the C1/C2 classification in 108 MPM tumor specimens with epithelioid and biphasic samples in both C1 and C2, and sarcomatoid samples only in C2.[74]

In 2016, 211 MPM transcriptomes were characterized using unsupervised consensus clustering, and 4 distinct molecular subtypes of MPM were identified: epithelioid, biphasic-E, biphasic-S, and sarcomatoid.[5] These subtypes were associated to a degree with the spectrum from epithelioid-to-sarcomatoid histology. The 62% of histologically epithelioid samples classified into the biphasic-E, biphasic-S, or sarcomatoid clusters showed significantly lower overall survival than those in the epithelioid cluster, indicating that epithelioid MPM can be distinguished into multiple different molecular groups. Differential expression analysis revealed that gene expression in the four clusters was related to the EMT process, consistent with previous findings.[74] Furthermore, a simple ratio of two genes, *CLDN15* and *VIM*, was able to significantly differentiate the samples in the four clusters. Four (*SETD2*, *TP53*, *NF2*, and *ULK2*) of the most significantly mutated genes showed mutation rates significantly different between cluster E and clusters BE, BS, and S.[75] Pathways implicated in this integrated analysis included histone methylation (consistent with previous findings, eg, Goto and colleagues,[34] 2009), Hippo, mTOR, RNA helicase, and p53 signaling.

In 2018, TCGA performed integrated analysis of 74 MPM tumors, including epigenetic, exomic, and transcriptomic profiles.[2] Integrative clustering performed using two separate algorithms (iCluster[76] and PARADIGM[77]) identified four distinct subtypes of MPM in each. These subtypes were highly concordant, particularly with respect to the more extreme clusters 1 and 4. These two clusters correlated significantly with survival even when controlling for histologic subtype and deletion of *CDKN2A*.[78] Cluster 1 was enriched for epithelioid histology, whereas cluster 4 was enriched for sarcomatoid tumors similarly to the Bueno cohort.[5] Genes associated with EMT transition were again differentially expressed between clusters. In addition, each cluster was characterized by a distinct immune profile. In particular, cluster 1 expressed the checkpoint inhibitor gene *VISTA* at high levels.

In an effort to deconvolute the signatures of epithelioid and sarcomatoid-like cell populations within bulk MPM samples, Blum and colleagues[8] performed a meta-analysis using several publicly available datasets.[5,72,74,79,80] Initially, they used transcriptome data to classify 63 MPM samples into four distinct clusters (C1A, C1B, C2A, and C2B). Next, they compared the expression profile of each cluster with the previously published expression-based cluster data. They identified two highly correlated molecular groups among all datasets corresponding with the most extreme epithelioid and sarcomatoid subtypes. The intermediary tumors, however, did not form distinguishable clusters, and therefore, the investigators suggest they reflect a continuum, or gradient, between epithelioid and sarcomatoid tumors. A panel of 150 common genes was used to generate 2 different scores, termed *E*-score and *S*-score, to determine the relative epithelioid-like and sarcomatoid-like molecular components present in individual tumors. Increased expression of *UPK3B*, *MSLN*, and *CLDN15* was correlated with *E*-score and *LOXL2* and *VIM* with the *S*-score. Pathway analysis revealed correlation of the *S*-score with EMT, TP53 signaling, cell cycle, angiogenesis, and immune checkpoints. The increasing sarcomatoid component identified by *S*-score was associated with worse outcomes in each series individually as well as in aggregate.[8]

Clinical applications of gene expression

MPM can be challenging to diagnose. Pleural plaques are not diagnostic for mesothelioma, and as previously described, the different MPM subtypes may be difficult to distinguish from other thoracic tumors on a histologic basis alone.[62] In addition, efforts to develop molecular predictors of clinical outcomes in MPM date back to the early 2000s, corresponding with the rapid proliferation of novel and cost-effective sequencing technologies, but few are regularly used in practice.[69,74,81–83]

The gene ratio-based method, developed by the authors' laboratory, is able to overcome the difficulty of validating large gene signatures and offers improved clinical applicability.[75,84] Developed by comparing expression profiles between patients with different clinicopathologic parameters, these tests can then predict tumor characteristics or clinical outcomes based on a small number of genes.[66,75] With respect to diagnosis, Gordon and colleagues[84] used 181 tissue samples to develop a 6-gene 3-ratio test to differentiate MPM from adenocarcinoma with 99% accuracy. De Rienzo and colleagues[85] used microarray data for 113 assorted MPM, non-MPM malignant, and benign samples to develop a sequential combination of binary gene-expression ratio tests in frozen tissues to discern MPM from other thoracic cancers, as well as to distinguish epithelioid from sarcomatoid MPM. Bruno and colleagues[86] used NanoString technology to develop and validate a diagnostic tool using 117 genes, of which 25 and 18 were upregulated and downregulated in MPM, respectively, as compared with benign mesothelial hyperplasia. Designed to work with small quantities of RNA, this test could be performed on formalin-fixed paraffin-embedded (FFPE) specimens.[86]

Similar strategies have been applied to prognosis. For example, a 4-gene 3-ratio (TM4SF1/PKM2, TM4SF1/ARHGDIA, COBLL1/ARHGDIA) test was developed to predict treatment-related outcome independent of histology based on real-time polymerase chain reaction expression data.[83,84] Although originally based on fresh-frozen tissue specimens, this score was later validated using FFPE tissue under Clinical Laboratory Improvement Amendments–approved guidelines in an independent multicenter cohort of MPM specimens.[85] It proved able to provide orthogonal risk information preoperatively, and, postoperatively, predict overall survival when combined with histopathologic information.

In addition to gene ratio tests, expression-based molecular subtype[74] and FAK protein expression[87] have been shown to correlate with sensitivity to the targeted agents verteporfin and defactinib, respectively. However, these and other targeted agents have not succeeded in clinical trials, and there are no current guidelines recommending their use.[20,29] Immunotherapy, although promising in several other cancer types, currently lacks biomarkers to predict efficacy in MPM because programmed death-ligand 1 (PD-L1) expression by IHC does not associate with treatment response.[88,89]

The immune microenvironment

Immunotherapy has expanded treatment options for tumors, such as melanoma and non–small cell lung cancer. Defining the immune microenvironment in MPM is an area of active investigation. In an early study, Burt and colleagues[90] demonstrated a significantly higher number of monocytes and tumor-infiltrating macrophages in nonepithelioid tumors. This study also found a significant association between higher monocyte counts and shorter survival. The checkpoint ligand PD-L1 is expressed in almost 40% of MPM tumors by RNA-seq, with significantly higher expression in sarcomatoid tumors.[5] Expression of CTLA-4, another checkpoint molecule, was found in varying levels in 56% of MPM tumor samples by IHC,

and higher in the epithelioid subtype.[91] In contrast, serum levels of soluble CTLA-4 were higher in patients with sarcomatoid disease as measured by enzyme-linked immunosorbent assay.[91]

Expression of immune mediators can drive tumor biology. An analysis of 87 advanced-stage (III or IV) MPM tumors combining IHC for PD-L1 and NanoString analysis for 805 genes revealed PD-L1 expression in 16% of samples with significantly higher PD-L1 expression in sarcomatoid and biphasic samples.[92] Using hierarchical clustering by gene expression, these investigators identified 3 subgroups of MPM: one with moderate T-cell effector gene expression but high B-cell gene expression (CD19, CD20); one with high PD-L1 expression and high T effector/T regulatory cell gene expression (including GZMA/GZMB, CXCL9, EOMES, FOXP3, ICOS, CTLA4); and one "immunologically ignorant" group with low expression of immune compartment-related genes but high stroma-related gene expression, including CTGF, DKK3, FN1, FAP, MMP2, and several genes encoding collagen subunits.[92] Taken together, these results suggest heterogeneity in the interaction between MPM and the immune microenvironment that warrants further exploration.

SUMMARY AND FUTURE DIRECTIONS

MPM is a rare and aggressive cancer caused by asbestos exposure in most cases. It is characterized by heterogeneity not only at the histologic but also at the molecular level. Its hallmarks include widespread chromosomal loss, mutations in tumor suppressor genes, such as BAP1, CDKN2A/2B, NF2, and TP53, and diverse transcriptomic phenotypes leading to several distinct molecular clusters. These clusters are defined at the extremes by epithelial and mesenchymal characteristics, with a histopathologic gradient stratifying the tumors in between. Multiple groups are working to develop predictive scores to classify individual tumors into these different subtypes, which have prognostic significance and may help guide choice of therapy.

Indeed, despite substantial advances in understanding the molecular biology of MPM, to date there have been relatively few changes in standard clinical practice based on these findings. MPM continues to present a diagnostic challenge and is often advanced at the time of detection. Histology remains the primary tool of prognostication in terms of overall survival and selection of therapeutic approach. Blunt, cytotoxic chemotherapy remains first-line systemic treatment for a nuanced, recalcitrant, and biologically complex disease.

Ongoing work in MPM molecular oncology will focus on deconvoluting the biological pathways involved in MPM tumorigenesis, growth, interaction with the tumor microenvironment, and response to therapy. Single-cell and single-nucleus transcriptomics have led to meaningful discoveries in several other cancers and offer the opportunity to define the contributions of individual tumor and immune/stromal cells to bulk tumor signatures. These techniques also provide a means to dissect intratumor heterogeneity and evaluate whether there are significant differences between malignant cells within an individual tumor, and how these might affect clinical outcomes.

Building on ever-expanding large datasets, deep learning and other advanced computational techniques are being used to integrate clinical, histopathologic, and molecular data to refine diagnostic approaches and identify new prognostic biomarkers (Courtiol and colleagues, 2019). New fields of study, such as proteomics and metabolomics, have yet to be incorporated into many of these analyses but show promise and merit further exploration (Sato and colleagues, 2018; Tomasetti and colleagues, 2019). Finally, the development of unique molecular signatures for individual tumors will help guide treatment selection and identify approaches to meaningfully improve patient survival on an individualized basis.

Clinics Care Points

- More than 80% of MPM is caused by asbestos exposure.
- MPM in patients with germline mutations is less aggressive and more chemotherapy-responsive than sporadic MPM, but these patients have a higher incidence of multiple other cancers.
- Gene ratio tests can be useful in distinguishing MPM from other thoracic disease processes, as well as for predicting response to treatment and overall survival.
- Transcriptomic and integrated multi-omic analyses can stratify MPM into distinct molecular clusters, which associate to a degree with histology and have independent implications for outcomes.
- Biomarkers to identify candidates for targeted therapy or immunotherapy in MPM are currently lacking.

DISCLOSURE

The authors disclose no potential conflicts of interest. Dr. Bueno reports research grants and clinical trials support from MedGenome, Roche, Verastem, Genentech, Merck, Gritstone, Epizyme, Siemens, NIH, and DOD. In addition, Dr. Bueno has 4 patents through the BWH (no royalties to date) and Equity in a new start-up company, Navigation Sciences.

REFERENCES

1. Broeckx G, Pauwels P. Malignant peritoneal mesothelioma: a review. Transl Lung Cancer Res 2018; 7(5):537–42.
2. Hmeljak J, Sanchez-Vega F, Hoadley KA, et al. Integrative molecular characterization of malignant pleural mesothelioma. Cancer Discov 2018;8(12): 1548–65.
3. Tischoff I, Neid M, Neumann V, et al. Pathohistological diagnosis and differential diagnosis. Recent Results Cancer Res 2011;189:57–78.
4. Vigneswaran WT, Kircheva DY, Ananthanarayanan V, et al. Amount of epithelioid differentiation is a predictor of survival in malignant pleural mesothelioma. Ann Thorac Surg 2017;103(3):962–6.
5. Bueno R, Stawiski EW, Goldstein LD, et al. Comprehensive genomic analysis of malignant pleural mesothelioma identifies recurrent mutations, gene fusions and splicing alterations. Nat Genet 2016; 48(4):407–16.
6. Yap TA, Aerts JG, Popat S, et al. Novel insights into mesothelioma biology and implications for therapy. Nat Rev Cancer 2017;17(8):475–88.
7. Oehl K, Vrugt B, Opitz I, et al. Heterogeneity in malignant pleural mesothelioma. Int J Mol Sci 2018; 19(6). https://doi.org/10.3390/ijms19061603.
8. Blum Y, Meiller C, Quetel L, et al. Dissecting heterogeneity in malignant pleural mesothelioma through histo-molecular gradients for clinical applications. Nat Commun 2019;10(1):1333.
9. Network NCC. Malignant pleural mesothelioma, version 2.2015. Secondary malignant pleural mesothelioma, version 2.2015. 2015. Available at: http://www.hts.org.gr/assets/files/omades_ergasias/cancer/NCCN%20guidelines%20Mesothelioma%202015.pdf. Accessed March 17, 2020.
10. Khan S, Gerber DE. Autoimmunity, checkpoint inhibitor therapy and immune-related adverse events: a review. Semin Cancer Biol 2019. https://doi.org/10.1016/j.semcancer.2019.06.012.
11. Gomez DR, Rimner A, Simone CB 2nd, et al. The use of radiation therapy for the treatment of malignant pleural mesothelioma: expert opinion from the National Cancer Institute Thoracic Malignancy Steering Committee, International Association for the Study of Lung Cancer, and Mesothelioma Applied Research Foundation. J Thorac Oncol 2019;14(7):1172–83.
12. Attanoos RL, Churg A, Galateau-Salle F, et al. Malignant mesothelioma and its non-asbestos causes. Arch Pathol Lab Med 2018;142(6):753–60.

13. Galani V, Varouktsi A, Papadatos SS, et al. The role of apoptosis defects in malignant mesothelioma pathogenesis with an impact on prognosis and treatment. Cancer Chemother Pharmacol 2019;84(2): 241–53.

14. Loomis D, Richardson DB, Elliott L. Quantitative relationships of exposure to chrysotile asbestos and mesothelioma mortality. Am J Ind Med 2019;62(6): 471–7.

15. Sun HH, Vaynblat A, Pass HI. Diagnosis and prognosis-review of biomarkers for mesothelioma. Ann Transl Med 2017;5(11):244.

16. Huang SX, Jaurand MC, Kamp DW, et al. Role of mutagenicity in asbestos fiber-induced carcinogenicity and other diseases. J Toxicol Environ Health B Crit Rev 2011;14(1–4):179–245.

17. Tomasetti M, Gaetani S, Monaco F, et al. Epigenetic regulation of miRNA expression in malignant mesothelioma: miRNAs as biomarkers of early diagnosis and therapy. Front Oncol 2019;9:1293.

18. Casalone E, Allione A, Viberti C, et al. DNA methylation profiling of asbestos-treated MeT5A cell line reveals novel pathways implicated in asbestos response. Arch Toxicol 2018;92(5):1785–95.

19. Nuvoli B, Camera E, Mastrofrancesco A, et al. Modulation of reactive oxygen species via ERK and STAT3 dependent signalling are involved in the response of mesothelioma cells to exemestane. Free Radic Biol Med 2018;115:266–77.

20. Zucali PA, Ceresoli GL, De Vincenzo F, et al. Advances in the biology of malignant pleural mesothelioma. Cancer Treat Rev 2011;37(7):543–58.

21. Pociask DA, Sime PJ, Brody AR. Asbestos-derived reactive oxygen species activate TGF-beta1. Lab Invest 2004;84(8):1013–23.

22. Kamp DW, Weitzman SA. The molecular basis of asbestos induced lung injury. Thorax 1999;54(7): 638–52.

23. Crovella S, Moura RR, Cappellani S, et al. A genetic variant of NLRP1 gene is associated with asbestos body burden in patients with malignant pleural mesothelioma. J Toxicol Environ Health A 2018;81(5): 98–105.

24. Celsi F, Crovella S, Moura RR, et al. Pleural mesothelioma and lung cancer: the role of asbestos exposure and genetic variants in selected iron metabolism and inflammation genes. J Toxicol Environ Health A 2019;82(20):1088–102.

25. Carbone M, Ly BH, Dodson RF, et al. Malignant mesothelioma: facts, myths, and hypotheses. J Cell Physiol 2012;227(1):44–58.

26. Jean D, Daubriac J, Le Pimpec-Barthes F, et al. Molecular changes in mesothelioma with an impact on prognosis and treatment. Arch Pathol Lab Med 2012;136(3):277–93.

27. Guo G, Chmielecki J, Goparaju C, et al. Whole-exome sequencing reveals frequent genetic alterations in BAP1, NF2, CDKN2A, and CUL1 in malignant pleural mesothelioma. Cancer Res 2015; 75(2):264–9.

28. Krismann M, Muller KM, Jaworska M, et al. Molecular cytogenetic differences between histological subtypes of malignant mesotheliomas: DNA cytometry and comparative genomic hybridization of 90 cases. J Pathol 2002;197(3):363–71.

29. Hylebos M, Van Camp G, van Meerbeeck JP, et al. The genetic landscape of malignant pleural mesothelioma: results from massively parallel sequencing. J Thorac Oncol 2016;11(10):1615–26.

30. Bott M, Brevet M, Taylor BS, et al. The nuclear deubiquitinase BAP1 is commonly inactivated by somatic mutations and 3p21.1 losses in malignant pleural mesothelioma. Nat Genet 2011;43(7): 668–72.

31. Lindholm PM, Salmenkivi K, Vauhkonen H, et al. Gene copy number analysis in malignant pleural mesothelioma using oligonucleotide array CGH. Cytogenet Genome Res 2007;119(1–2):46–52.

32. Borczuk AC, Pei J, Taub RN, et al. Genome-wide analysis of abdominal and pleural malignant mesothelioma with DNA arrays reveals both common and distinct regions of copy number alteration. Cancer Biol Ther 2016;17(3):328–35.

33. Tsou JA, Galler JS, Wali A, et al. DNA methylation profile of 28 potential marker loci in malignant mesothelioma. Lung Cancer 2007;58(2):220–30.

34. Goto Y, Shinjo K, Kondo Y, et al. Epigenetic profiles distinguish malignant pleural mesothelioma from lung adenocarcinoma. Cancer Res 2009;69(23): 9073–82.

35. Christensen BC, Houseman EA, Godleski JJ, et al. Epigenetic profiles distinguish pleural mesothelioma from normal pleura and predict lung asbestos burden and clinical outcome. Cancer Res 2009; 69(1):227–34.

36. Laszlo V, Hoda MA, Garay T, et al. Epigenetic downregulation of integrin alpha7 increases migratory potential and confers poor prognosis in malignant pleural mesothelioma. J Pathol 2015;237(2):203–14.

37. Christensen BC, Houseman EA, Poage GM, et al. Integrated profiling reveals a global correlation between epigenetic and genetic alterations in mesothelioma. Cancer Res 2010;70(14):5686–94.

38. Reid G, Johnson TG, van Zandwijk N. Manipulating microRNAs for the treatment of malignant pleural mesothelioma: past, present and future. Front Oncol 2020;10:105.

39. Quetel L, Tranchant R, Meiller C, et al. Abstract 112: genetic alterations in molecular tumor subgroups of malignant pleural mesothelioma. Cancer Res 2016; 76(14 Supplement):112.

40. Cigognetti M, Lonardi S, Fisogni S, et al. BAP1 (BRCA1-associated protein 1) is a highly specific marker for differentiating mesothelioma from

reactive mesothelial proliferations. Mod Pathol 2015; 28(8):1043–57.

41. Ladanyi M, Robinson BW, Campbell PJ, et al. The TCGA malignant pleural mesothelioma (MPM) project: VISTA expression and delineation of a novel clinical-molecular subtype of MPM. J Clin Oncol 2018;36(15_suppl):8516.

42. Carbone M, Yang H, Pass HI, et al. BAP1 and cancer. Nat Rev Cancer 2013;13(3):153–9.

43. Yu H, Pak H, Hammond-Martel I, et al. Tumor suppressor and deubiquitinase BAP1 promotes DNA double-strand break repair. Proc Natl Acad Sci U S A 2014;111(1):285–90.

44. De Rienzo A, Archer MA, Yeap BY, et al. Gender-specific molecular and clinical features underlie malignant pleural mesothelioma. Cancer Res 2016; 76(2):319–28.

45. Bononi A, Giorgi C, Patergnani S, et al. BAP1 regulates IP3R3-mediated Ca(2+) flux to mitochondria suppressing cell transformation. Nature 2017; 546(7659):549–53.

46. McCambridge AJ, Napolitano A, Mansfield AS, et al. Progress in the management of malignant pleural mesothelioma in 2017. J Thorac Oncol 2018;13(5):606–23.

47. Righi L, Duregon E, Vatrano S, et al. BRCA1-associated protein 1 (BAP1) immunohistochemical expression as a diagnostic tool in malignant pleural mesothelioma classification: a large retrospective study. J Thorac Oncol 2016;11(11): 2006–17.

48. LaFave LM, Beguelin W, Koche R, et al. Loss of BAP1 function leads to EZH2-dependent transformation. Nat Med 2015;21(11):1344–9.

49. Sage AP, Martinez VD, Minatel BC, et al. Genomics and epigenetics of malignant mesothelioma. High Throughput 2018;7(3). https://doi.org/10.3390/ht7030020.

50. Jean D, Jaurand M-C. Causes and pathophysiology of malignant pleural mesothelioma. Lung Cancer Management 2015;4(5):219–29.

51. Tranchant R, Quetel L, Tallet A, et al. Co-occurring mutations of tumor suppressor genes, LATS2 and NF2, in malignant pleural mesothelioma. Clin Cancer Res 2017;23(12):3191–202.

52. Panou V, Gadiraju M, Wolin A, et al. Frequency of germline mutations in cancer susceptibility genes in malignant mesothelioma. J Clin Oncol 2018; 36(28):2863–71.

53. Hassan R, Morrow B, Thomas A, et al. Inherited predisposition to malignant mesothelioma and overall survival following platinum chemotherapy. Proc Natl Acad Sci U S A 2019;116(18):9008–13.

54. Guo R, DuBoff M, Jayakumaran G, et al. Novel germline mutations in DNA damage repair in patients with malignant pleural mesotheliomas. J Thorac Oncol 2019. https://doi.org/10.1016/j.jtho.2019.12.111.

55. Carbone M, Adusumilli PS, Alexander HR Jr, et al. Mesothelioma: scientific clues for prevention, diagnosis, and therapy. CA Cancer J Clin 2019;69(5): 402–29.

56. Testa JR, Cheung M, Pei J, et al. Germline BAP1 mutations predispose to malignant mesothelioma. Nat Genet 2011;43(10):1022–5.

57. Luchini C, Veronese N, Yachida S, et al. Different prognostic roles of tumor suppressor gene BAP1 in cancer: a systematic review with meta-analysis. Genes Chromosomes Cancer 2016; 55(10):741–9.

58. Carbone M, Ferris LK, Baumann F, et al. BAP1 cancer syndrome: malignant mesothelioma, uveal and cutaneous melanoma, and MBAITs. J Transl Med 2012;10:179.

59. Walpole S, Pritchard AL, Cebulla CM, et al. Comprehensive study of the clinical phenotype of germline BAP1 variant-carrying families worldwide. J Natl Cancer Inst 2018;110(12):1328–41.

60. Pulford E, Huilgol K, Moffat D, et al. Malignant mesothelioma, BAP1 immunohistochemistry, and VEGFA: does BAP1 have potential for early diagnosis and assessment of prognosis? Dis Markers 2017;2017: 1310478.

61. Parrotta R, Okonska A, Ronner M, et al. A novel BRCA1-associated protein-1 isoform affects response of mesothelioma cells to drugs impairing BRCA1-mediated DNA repair. J Thorac Oncol 2017;12(8):1309–19.

62. Ray M, Kindler HL. Malignant pleural mesothelioma: an update on biomarkers and treatment. Chest 2009;136(3):888–96.

63. Churg A, Nabeshima K, Ali G, et al. Highlights of the 14th International Mesothelioma Interest Group meeting: pathologic separation of benign from malignant mesothelial proliferations and histologic/molecular analysis of malignant mesothelioma subtypes. Lung Cancer 2018;124:95–101.

64. Galateau Salle F, Le Stang N, Nicholson AG, et al. New insights on diagnostic reproducibility of biphasic mesotheliomas: a multi-institutional evaluation by the International Mesothelioma Panel from the MESOPATH reference center. J Thorac Oncol 2018;13(8):1189–203.

65. Uhlen M, Zhang C, Lee S, et al. A pathology atlas of the human cancer transcriptome. Science 2017;357: 6352.

66. Gordon GJ. Transcriptional profiling of mesothelioma using microarrays. Lung Cancer 2005; 49(Suppl 1):S99–103.

67. Rihn BH, Mohr S, McDowell SA, et al. Differential gene expression in mesothelioma. FEBS Lett 2000; 480(2–3):95–100.

68. Singhal S, Wiewrodt R, Malden LD, et al. Gene expression profiling of malignant mesothelioma. Clin Cancer Res 2003;9(8):3080–97.

69. Pass HI, Liu Z, Wali A, et al. Gene expression profiles predict survival and progression of pleural mesothelioma. Clin Cancer Res 2004;10(3):849–59.

70. Guled M, Lahti L, Lindholm PM, et al. CDKN2A, NF2, and JUN are dysregulated among other genes by miRNAs in malignant mesothelioma -a miRNA microarray analysis. Genes Chromosomes Cancer 2009; 48(7):615–23.

71. Melaiu O, Cristaudo A, Melissari E, et al. A review of transcriptome studies combined with data mining reveals novel potential markers of malignant pleural mesothelioma. Mutat Res 2012;750(2):132–40.

72. Gordon GJ, Rockwell GN, Jensen RV, et al. Identification of novel candidate oncogenes and tumor suppressors in malignant pleural mesothelioma using large-scale transcriptional profiling. Am J Pathol 2005;166(6):1827–40.

73. Suraokar MB, Nunez MI, Diao L, et al. Expression profiling stratifies mesothelioma tumors and signifies deregulation of spindle checkpoint pathway and microtubule network with therapeutic implications. Ann Oncol 2014;25(6):1184–92.

74. de Reynies A, Jaurand MC, Renier A, et al. Molecular classification of malignant pleural mesothelioma: identification of a poor prognosis subgroup linked to the epithelial-to-mesenchymal transition. Clin Cancer Res 2014;20(5):1323–34.

75. De Rienzo A, Richards WG, Bueno R. Gene signature of malignant pleural mesothelioma. In: Testa JR, editor. Asbestos and mesothelioma. 2017. p. 197–209.

76. Shen R, Olshen AB, Ladanyi M. Integrative clustering of multiple genomic data types using a joint latent variable model with application to breast and lung cancer subtype analysis. Bioinformatics 2009; 25(22):2906–12.

77. Vaske CJ, Benz SC, Sanborn JZ, et al. Inference of patient-specific pathway activities from multidimensional cancer genomics data using PARADIGM. Bioinformatics 2010;26(12):i237–45.

78. Dacic S, Kothmaier H, Land S, et al. Prognostic significance of p16/cdkn2a loss in pleural malignant mesotheliomas. Virchows Arch 2008;453(6):627–35.

79. Lopez-Rios F, Chuai S, Flores R, et al. Global gene expression profiling of pleural mesotheliomas: overexpression of aurora kinases and P16/CDKN2A deletion as prognostic factors and critical evaluation of microarray-based prognostic prediction. Cancer Res 2006;66(6):2970–9.

80. Center BITGDA. Analysis-ready standardized TCGA data from Broad GDAC Firehose stddata__2015_ 06_01run. Boston (MA): Harvard BIoMa; 2015.

81. Gordon GJ, Jensen RV, Hsiao LL, et al. Using gene expression ratios to predict outcome among patients with mesothelioma. J Natl Cancer Inst 2003; 95(8):598–605.

82. Gordon GJ, Rockwell GN, Godfrey PA, et al. Validation of genomics-based prognostic tests in malignant pleural mesothelioma. Clin Cancer Res 2005; 11(12):4406–14.

83. Gordon GJ, Dong L, Yeap BY, et al. Four-gene expression ratio test for survival in patients undergoing surgery for mesothelioma. J Natl Cancer Inst 2009;101(9):678–86.

84. Gordon GJ, Jensen RV, Hsiao LL, et al. Translation of microarray data into clinically relevant cancer diagnostic tests using gene expression ratios in lung cancer and mesothelioma. Cancer Res 2002; 62(17):4963–7.

85. De Rienzo A, Cook RW, Wilkinson J, et al. Validation of a gene expression test for mesothelioma prognosis in formalin-fixed paraffin-embedded tissues. J Mol Diagn 2017;19(1):65–71.

86. Bruno R, Ali G, Giannini R, et al. Malignant pleural mesothelioma and mesothelial hyperplasia: a new molecular tool for the differential diagnosis. Oncotarget 2017;8(2):2758–70.

87. Tranchant R, Quetel L, Montagne F, et al. Assessment of signaling pathway inhibitors and identification of predictive biomarkers in malignant pleural mesothelioma. Lung Cancer 2018;126:15–24.

88. Nowak AK, McDonnell A, Cook A. Immune checkpoint inhibition for the treatment of mesothelioma. Expert Opin Biol Ther 2019;19(7):697–706.

89. Alley EW, Lopez J, Santoro A, et al. Clinical safety and activity of pembrolizumab in patients with malignant pleural mesothelioma (KEYNOTE-028): preliminary results from a non-randomised, open-label, phase 1b trial. Lancet Oncol 2017;18(5):623–30.

90. Burt BM, Rodig SJ, Tilleman TR, et al. Circulating and tumor-infiltrating myeloid cells predict survival in human pleural mesothelioma. Cancer 2011; 117(22):5234–44.

91. Roncella S, Laurent S, Fontana V, et al. CTLA-4 in mesothelioma patients: tissue expression, body fluid levels and possible relevance as a prognostic factor. Cancer Immunol Immunother 2016;65(8):909–17.

92. Patil NS, Righi L, Koeppen H, et al. Molecular and histopathological characterization of the tumor immune microenvironment in advanced stage of malignant pleural mesothelioma. J Thorac Oncol 2018;13(1):124–33.

Mesothelioma Biomarkers
Discovery in Search of Validation

Harvey I. Pass, MD[a,*], Marjan Alimi, MD[b], Michele Carbone, MD, PhD[c], Haining Yang, PhD[c], Chandra M. Goparaju, PhD[b]

KEYWORDS

- Mesothelioma • Biomarkers • Asbestos • Prognosis • Diagnosis

KEY POINTS

- Malignant pleural mesothelioma (MPM) is an asbestos-related neoplasm that can only be treated successfully when correctly diagnosed and treated in early stages.
- The asbestos-exposed population serves as a high-risk group that could benefit from sensitive and specific blood- or tissue-based biomarkers.
- The literature of the last 20 years is reviewed to comment on the most promising of the blood- and tissue-based biomarkers.
- SMRP remains as the only validated blood-based biomarker with diagnostic, monitoring, and prognostic value. Other biomarkers, such as calretinin, fibulin 3, and HMGB1, remain under study and need international validation trials with large cohorts of cases and controls to demonstrate any utility.
- To strengthen the development and testing of MPM biomarkers, cohorts for validation must be established by enlisting collaborations from all over the world.

INTRODUCTION

Malignant pleural mesothelioma (MPM) is an aggressive type of cancer originating from the serosal surface of the lungs, and is thought to be primarily caused by asbestos exposure and less commonly due to exposure to high-dose radiation and certain mineral fibers. The role of SV40 infection continues to be controversial.[1–8] Although the incidence is low and estimated around 3200 cases per year in the US, the mortality is particularly high due to its aggressiveness and diagnosis at late stages.[9–11] There is approximately 20 to 40 years latency between the time of exposure and clinical diagnosis, during which chronic asbestos exposure creates a persistent inflammatory response (the inflammasome). This response has a myriad of actions on cytokines and reactive oxygen species (ROS) that potentially lead to MPM carcinogenesis pathway.[12–16] Data from various studies strongly support that MPM has a low mutation burden and the most frequently mutated genes involved in MPM pathogenesis are tumor suppressor genes, including BAP1, NF2, and CDKN2A.[17–21]

Histologically, MPM is classified into 3 main different subtypes. The epithelioid subtype characterizes the most common and least aggressive type, consisting approximately of 70% of MPMs. The sarcomatoid subtype is the most aggressive type and is highly resistant to chemotherapy and associated with the worst prognosis. The biphasic subtype denotes an intermediate type corresponding to a transition between the other 2 histologic subtypes.[1,9] Kadota and colleagues[22] reported the median survival length for epithelioid, biphasic and sarcomatoid subtypes to be 16.2, 7.0, and 3.8 months, respectively.

[a] Research, Department of Cardiothoracic Surgery, General Thoracic Surgery, NYU Langone Medical Center, 530 First Avenue, 9V, New York, NY 10016, USA; [b] Department of Cardiothoracic Surgery, NYU Langone Medical Center, 530 First Avenue, 9V, New York, NY 10016, USA; [c] Department of Thoracic Oncology, John A. Burns School of Medicine, University of Hawaii Cancer Center, 701 Ilalo Street, Room 437, Honolulu, HI 96813, USA
* Corresponding author.
E-mail address: harvey.pass@nyumc.org

Thorac Surg Clin 30 (2020) 395–423
https://doi.org/10.1016/j.thorsurg.2020.08.001
1547-4127/20/© 2020 Elsevier Inc. All rights reserved.

Early-stage MPM is associated with significantly better outcome and overall survival (OS) compared with late-stage disease that is minimally responsive to aggressive multimodality therapy with surgery, chemotherapy, and radiation therapy.[1,23–28] Unfortunately, the former group constitutes only 5% of the patients with MPM and, therefore, the average survival is about 13 months in all patients.[9] Given that early diagnosis is of critical importance in improving the outcome and chance for cure, extensive research has focused on identifying optimal screening strategies for populations at risk.[29,30] This is particularly important since, contrary to common assumption, asbestos continues to be used worldwide and thus MPM rate is not expected to decrease. An optimal screening test is noninvasive, easily accessible, concomitantly highly sensitive and specific (highly accurate), and ideally cost-effective. Although imaging methods are mostly noninvasive, current modalities, including computed tomography scans, are found to be ineffective and nonspecific in early diagnosis of MPM.[31] Pleural biopsy remains the diagnostic method of choice for MPM, but introduces potential morbidity and cost.[32] As a result, there is a critical need for effective noninvasive screening methods for high-risk, asbestos-exposed populations to assist in diagnosis and treatment of patients with MPM at earlier stages. Accordingly, over the past 2 decades, biomarkers have gained a high level of attention and have been extensively studied (**Table 1**).

Mesothelin, Soluble Mesothelin-Related Proteins, and Megakaryocyte Potentiating Factor

Mesothelin (MSLN), a protein believed to have a role in cellular adhesion, was the first biomarker studied for MPM and was originally discovered and described by Chang and Pastan.[33] After initial translation into a precursor protein, MSLN and megakaryocyte potentiating factor (MPF) are formed by cleavage of the preprotein into 41K and 30K molecules, respectively.[34–36] MSLN was found to activate the nuclear factor κB pathway, thereby promoting cell proliferation and survival.[37] Although low levels of MSLN are produced by normal mesothelial cells, overexpression has been seen in certain cancers, including MPM, pancreatic adenocarcinoma, and ovarian and lung cancers.[38,39] Soluble mesothelin-related peptide (SMRP) is a soluble form of MSLN released by tumor cells into the circulation and is the only Food and Drug Administration-approved biomarker for diagnosis of MPM.[40,41] Following the original description of SMRP by Hellstrom and colleagues,[34] it was commercialized by Fujirebio.[35,42] The diagnostic value of SMRP in MPM was first studied and described by Robinson and colleagues.[35] After technical and clinical validation of the MESOMARK assay in serum and pleural effusion (PE) of North American population,[42,43] the serum level of SMRP was found to be capable of differentiating patients with MPM from asbestos-exposed and asbestos-unexposed individuals, as well as those with benign pleural diseases.[44–47] These early studies were followed by an international blinded trial of MESOMARK levels in 165 MPM cases and 652 asbestos-exposed controls, where serum samples from Australia and North America were independently measured by Fujirebio and the UCLA Early Detection Research Laboratory Biomarker Reference Laboratory. Discrimination between cases and controls was validated at both sites with very similar sensitivity and specificity, as seen in **Fig. 1**, and later studies confirmed these findings.[42] In a systematic review and meta-analysis of SMRP for MPM discrimination, Luo and colleagues[48] pooled data from 12 studies with 717 patients with MPM and 2851 controls (including healthy individuals and patients with non-MPM diseases) and found 64% sensitivity and 89% specificity for serum SMRPs in diagnosis of MPM. On the other hand, Hollevoet and colleagues[49] performed a meta-analysis of 16 studies with 1026 MPM cases and 4491 controls that revealed 32% sensitivity and 95% specificity for MSLN in diagnosis of MPM. Other studies suggested the potential capability of MSLN in discriminating between MPM and pleural metastases.[42,45,47]

Utility of SMRP in screening for MPM in high-risk asbestos-exposed population was further explored in a subset of patients from Beta-Carotene and Retinol Efficacy Trial (CARET), a large study in which the potential role of vitamin supplementation in chemoprevention of lung cancer was investigated. A total of 4060 heavily asbestos-exposed US men were followed for 9 to 17 years, among whom 49 developed MPM while on the CARET. Forty-nine MPM cases and 96 matched controls were studied to elucidate whether SMRP was able to predict development of MPM years before the clinical presentation. Accordingly, serum markers were measured blindly at 2 separate sites, and unsurprisingly showed an overall ROC (receiver operating curve) AUC (area under the curve) of 0.604 (95% CI, 0.489–0.699), likely given that MPM markers may not be increased several years before the diagnosis. Conversely, serum SMRP levels measured less than a year before diagnosis had an AUC of

Table 1
Summary of major biomarkers for diagnosis of MPM

Biomarker	Author, Year	N (MPM/Total)	Compared Groups	Method	Results	Conclusion
Mesothelin	Creaney et al,[64] 2014	82/153	Non-MPM malignant, benign	Plasma, pleural fluid; ELISA (mesothelin and fibulin-3)	Mesothelin showed high diagnostic accuracy for MPM Plasma AUC, 0.822 Pleural AUC, 0.815	Mesothelin is a superior diagnostic biomarker for MPM compared with fibulin-3
	Bayram et al,[239] 2014	24/546	Pleural plaques, healthy asbestos exposed, healthy unexposed	Serum; ELISA (mesothelin and osteopontin)	Mesothelin level was independently associated with MPM, age, smoking pack years, and BMI. It differentiated MPM from other groups Sensitivity, 58% Specificity, 83%	Combination of mesothelin with osteopontin provides higher diagnostic accuracy
	Creaney et al,[40] 2013	66/213	Other malignant, benign, asbestos exposed, healthy, kidney disease	Pleural fluid, serum ELISA	Serum and pleural mesothelin was increased in MPM compared with all controls Serum AUC, 0.829 Pleural AUC, 0.928	Mesothelin conveys diagnostic accuracy in both serum and pleural fluid (equivalent to MPF
	Hollevoet et al,[49] 2012	1026/5517	Non-MPM (various controls)	Review and meta-analysis	At 95% specificity, sensitivity was 32% AUC, 0.77 (95% CI, 0.73–0.81)	Mesothelin is highly specific for diagnosis of MPM, but lacks adequate sensitivity for screening
SMRP	Burt et al,[54] 2017	102	—	Serum, ELISA	Percentage of change in serial postop SMRP values at cutoff of 48% was highly predictive of disease recurrence AUC, 0.96	Serial SMRP level measurements can aid in detection of recurrence after resection of MPM
	Demir et al,[98] 2016	42/131	Asbestos exposed, healthy	Serum (various markers, including SMRP, thioredoxin-1 (TRX) EGFR, mesothelin, syndecan-1, fibulin-3)	SMRP showed graded increase: control-asbestos-MPM, and was able to distinguish MPM from other groups AUC, 0.86	SMRP and TRX provide better diagnostic accuracy than EGFR, mesothelin, syndecan-1, fibulin-3

(continued on next page)

Table 1
(continued)

Biomarker	Author, Year	N (MPM/Total)	Compared Groups	Method	Results	Conclusion
	Santarelli et al,[144] 2015	45/188	Asbestos exposed, healthy	Serum (various markers, including SMRP, miR-126 and methylated thrombomodulin [Met-TM])	Combination of SMRP, miR-126 and Met-TM has higher diagnostic accuracy compared with isolated SMRP AUC, 0.857 vs 0.818	Combined panel of SMRP with other biomarkers improves diagnostic value of SMRP for MPM
	Filiberti et al,[50] 2013	–/1704	Asbestos-related pleural lesions, benign, healthy	Blood, ELISA	Predictors of increased SMRP were age >57, current smoking, BMI <25, positive anamnesis for cancer and for asbestos-related pleural lesions	SMRP is a candidate marker predictive of MPM
	Hollevoet et al,[55] 2011	215(->179->137)	–	Serum, ELISA	SMRP and MPF showed a high intraclass correlation Single biomarker measurement and fixed threshold are suboptimal in screening	Biomarker-based screening approach can be improved by incorporation of serial measurements and adjustment for age and GFR
	Hollevoet et al,[69] 2010	85/507	Healthy, healthy asbestos-exposed, benign asbestos-related disease, benign respiratory disease, lung cancer	Serum; MesoMark ELISAs (MPF and SMRP)	SMRP (and MPF) levels were significantly higher in MPM compared with all other groups AUC for SMRP, 0.871 (AUC for MPF, 0.849)	SMRP has been shown to be a highly performant MPM biomarker
	Luo et al,[48] 2010	717/3568	Non-MPM (various controls)	Review and meta-analysis	SMRPs had a pooled sensitivity of 0.64 (95% CI, 0.61–0.68), specificity of 0.89 (95% CI, 0.88–0.90), positive likelihood ratio of 7.10 (95% CI, 4.44–11.35), negative likelihood ratio of 0.39 (95% CI, 0.31–0.48), and diagnostic odds ratio of 19.35 (95% CI, 10.95–34.17)	Serum SMRP level is a candidate biomarker for diagnosis of MPM
	Rodriguez Portal et al,[46] 2009	36/362	Healthy, asbestos exposed without pleural disease, asbestos exposed with benign pleural disease	Serum; ELISA	Serum SMRP levels were higher in MPM compared with other groups AUC, 0.75	Serum SMRP level is a potential biomarker for diagnosis of MPM

	Reference	No.	Population	Sample; Method	Results	Conclusions
	Pass et al,[43] 2008	90/326	Lung cancer, asbestos exposed	Serum, pleural effusion; MesoMark ELISAs	Serum SMRP levels were higher in MPM compared with asbestos exposed AUC, 0.81. SMRP levels were higher in stages 2–4 MPM compared with stage 1 MPM	Serum and pleural SMRP levels can be used in screening asbestos-exposed individuals
	Pass et al,[53] 2008	30/85	—	MesoMark ELISAs (response to therapy with a copper reducing agent tetrathiomolybdate, assessed by target ceruloplasmin levels and VGEF levels)	SMRP levels decreased immediately postsurgery and increased over time during progression of disease	SMRPs can have a role in monitoring posttreatment patients with MPM
	Park et al,[51] 2008	–/538	—	Serum; ELISA	Mean SMRP in healthy subjects was significantly lower than in subjects with pleural plaques	SMRP has a high false positive rate and seems unlikely to prove useful in screening for MPM
	Scherpereel et al,[45] 2006	74/137	Pleural metastasis of carcinomas, benign pleural lesions associated with asbestos exposure	Serum, pleural effusion; ELISA	SMRP level was higher in MPM than in metastasis or benign lesions. Serum AUC for differentiating MPM and benign, 0.872. Serum AUC for differentiating MPM and metastasis, 0.693. Pleural AUC for differentiating MPM and benign, 0.831. Pleural AUC for differentiating MPM and metastasis, 0.793	Serum and pleural SMRP levels can be used as biomarkers in diagnosis of MPM
	Robinson et al,[35] 2003	44/272	Healthy, asbestos exposed, other inflammatory or malignant lung and pleural diseases	Serum; ELISA	SMRP levels were increased in the vast majority of patients with MPM. Increased SMRP levels in asbestos-exposed individuals may predict development of MPM. SMRP concentrations correlated with tumor size and progression	SMRP level can be helpful in diagnosis of MPM and screening of asbestos-exposed high-risk individuals
MPF	Creaney et al,[40] 2013	66/213	Other malignant, benign, asbestos exposed, healthy, kidney disease	Pleural fluid, serum; ELISA	Serum and pleural MPF were increased in MPM compared with all controls Serum AUC, 0.813 Pleural AUC, 0.945	MPF conveys diagnostic accuracy in both serum and pleural fluid (equivalent to mesothelin)
	Hollevoet et al,[69] 2010	85/507	Healthy, healthy asbestos-exposed, benign asbestos-related disease, benign respiratory disease, lung cancer	Serum; MesoMark ELISAs (MPF and SMRP)	MPF (and SMRP) levels were significantly higher in MPM compared with all other groups AUC for MPF, 0.849 (AUC for SMRP, 0.871)	MPF is validated as a highly performant MPM biomarker (equivalent to SMRP)

(continued on next page)

Table 1
(continued)

Biomarker	Author, Year	N (MPM/Total)	Compared Groups	Method	Results	Conclusion
Osteopontin	Onda et al,[68] 2006	56/126	Healthy	Serum, ELISA (MPF and SMRP)	MPF level was increased in 91% of patients with MPM compared with healthy controls	MPF can aid in diagnosis of MPM
	Hu et al,[89] 2014	360/906	Non-MPM (various controls)	Review and meta-analysis	Osteopontin pooled diagnostic sensitivity and specificity for MPM was 0.65 and 0.81, respectively AUC, 0.83	Osteopontin is an effective biomarker for MPM diagnosis
	Bayram et al,[239] 2014	24/546	Pleural plaques, healthy asbestos exposed, healthy unexposed	Serum; ELISA (osteopontin and mesothelin)	Osteopontin level was independently associated with MPM, age, smoking pack years, and BMI. It was able to differentiate MPM from other groups Sensitivity, 75% Specificity, 86%	Combination of osteopontin with mesothelin provides higher diagnostic accuracy
	Felten et al,[82] 2014	–/2262	Formerly asbestos exposed, unknown history of asbestos exposure, nonasbestos exposed	Blood; commercial ELISA (osteopontin and mesothelin)	Osteopontin rise was associated with age	Age effects on biomarkers need to be taken into account
	Creaney et al,[88] 2011	66/176	Nonmalignant asbestos-related lung or pleural disease, other benign pleural and lung diseases, lung cancer	Serum and plasma (osteopontin and mesothelin)	Serum and plasma osteopontin levels were significantly higher in patients with MPM compared with benign lung and pleural disease AUC for serum, 0.639 AUC for plasma, 0.763 Combining the serum mesothelin and plasma osteopontin did not increase AUC	Plasma osteopontin has a superior diagnostic accuracy to serum osteopontin
	Cristaudo et al,[84] 2011	31/235	Healthy, benign respiratory disease	Plasma; ELISA (plasma osteopontin and serum SMRP)	Plasma osteopontin level was significantly higher in patients with MPM compared with other groups AUC, 0.795	Combined osteopontin and SMRP panel provides a high accuracy for diagnosis of MPM AUC, 0.873
	Rai et al,[86] 2010	205/286	Healthy, nonmesothelioma other patients with cancer	Plasma; ELISA (plasma osteopontin and serum SMRP)	Osteopontin level was significantly higher in patients with MPM compared with other groups AUC for osteopontin, 0.68 AUC for SMRP, 0.89	Both osteopontin and SMRP can be used as biomarkers in diagnosis of MPM

Biomarker	Study	Cases/Controls	Control Group	Sample; Method	Results	Conclusion
	Grigoriu et al,[61] 2007	96/284	Pleural metastases of various carcinomas, benign pleural lesions associated with asbestos exposure, asbestos-exposed healthy	Serum, pleural fluid; ELISA	Osteopontin was able to distinguish MPM from healthy asbestos exposed (AUC, 0.724); however, could not distinguish between MPM and pleural metastatic carcinoma or benign pleural lesions associated with asbestos exposure	Insufficient specificity limits osteopontin utility as a diagnostic marker
	Pass et al,[80] 2005	76/190	Asbestos-related nonmalignant pulmonary disease, healthy nonasbestos exposed	Serum; ELISA	Serum osteopontin level was able to distinguish patients with MPM from asbestos-exposed patients with high sensitivity and specificity AUC, 0.888	Serum osteopontin can be used a biomarker for diagnosis of MPM in asbestos-exposed individuals
Fibulin-3	Pei et al,[103] 2017	468/1132	Non-MPM (various controls)	Review and meta-analysis	Serum fibulin-3 level had a pooled sensitivity of 62% (95% CI, 45%–77%) and specificity of 82% (95% CI, 73%–89%) for in diagnosis of MPM AUC, 0.81	Fibulin-3 has a relatively high diagnostic efficacy for identification of MPM
	Napolitano et al,[183] 2016	22/100	Asbestos exposed, benign effusion, other malignant effusion, healthy	Serum; ELISA	Fibulin-3 was able to distinguish MPM with high accuracy AUC, 0.959. Combining fibulin-3 with HMGB1 resulted in higher sensitivity, and specificity for differentiating MPM	Combined panel of fibulin-3 and HMGB1, is effective in diagnosis of MPM
	Kaya et al,[100] 2015	43/83	Healthy	Serum; ELISA	Serum fibulin-3 level was significantly higher in patients with MPM compared with controls AUC, 0.976	Serum fibulin-3 is a useful biomarker for diagnosis of MPM
	Creaney et al,[64] 2014	82/153	Non-MM malignant, benign	Plasma, pleural fluid; ELISA (fibulin-3 and mesothelin)	Fibulin-3 showed lower diagnostic accuracy for MPM compared with mesothelin. Plasma AUC, 0.671. Pleural AUC, 0.588	Pleural fibulin-3 is an independent prognostic factor for survival; not as effective for diagnosis

(continued on next page)

Table 1
(continued)

Biomarker	Author, Year	N (MPM/Total)	Compared Groups	Method	Results	Conclusion
	Pass et al,[96] 2012	92/364	Asbestos exposed without cancer, patients with effusions not due to mesothelioma, healthy controls	Plasma, pleural fluid; ELISA	Plasma fibulin-3 was significantly higher in MPM compared with asbestos-exposed persons without mesothelioma AUC, 0.99 Effusion fibulin-3 was significantly higher in MPM compared with effusions not due to mesothelioma AUC, 0.93	Plasma fibulin-3 can aid in diagnosis of MPM in asbestos-exposed individuals Pleural fibulin-3 can better aid in differentiation of MPM from other pathologies
Proteomic	Ostroff et al,[107] 2012	117/259	Asbestos exposed	Serum; SOMAmer proteomic technology	The identified 13-marker SOMAmer panel was able to accurately distinguish patients with MPM AUC, 0.99 It showed better performance than mesothelin Sensitivity correlated with pathologic stage	SOMAmer biomarker panel provides a strong surveillance method for diagnosis of MPM in population at risk
Glycomic	Cerciello et al,[111] 2013	23/75	Healthy, non-small cell lung cancer (NSCLC)	Serum; selected reaction monitoring (SRM) assay technology (glycopeptides and mesothelin)	The identified 7-glycopeptide signature discriminated patients with MPM from healthy donors (AUC, 0.94), but not from patients with NSCLC	Glycomic technology can provide a helpful diagnostic tool for MPM in adjunction with other biomarkers
miRNAs	Sun et al,[150] 2018	93/146	Asbestos exposed	Serum; HTG EdgeSeq miRNA whole transcriptome assay	An identified 7-miRNA signature was able to differentiate MPMs from asbestos exposed AUC, 0.953	The 7-miRNA signature can aid in early diagnosis of MPM
	Bononi et al,[151] 2016	10/30	Asbestos-exposed workers; healthy	Serum; microarray, real-time qPCR	miR-197-3p, miR 1281, miR-32-3p upregulated in MPM	Distinct mRNAs are potential new biomarkers for diagnosis of MPM
	Santarelli et al,[143] 2015	45/188	Asbestos exposed, healthy	Serum (various markers, including miR-126, SMRP, and Met-TM)	Combination of miR-126, SMRP, and Met-TM has higher diagnostic accuracy compared to isolated SMRP AUC, 0.857 vs 0.818	Combined 3 biomarker panel including miR-126, provides high diagnostic accuracy for MPM
	Andersen et al,[148] 2014	45/76	Reactive mesothelial proliferations (RMP)	Tissue Real-time qPCR, formaldehyde-fixed paraffin embedded preoperative biopsy samples	A 4 miRNA group including miR-126, miR-143, miR145, miR-652 was able to accurately differentiate MPM AUC, 0.96	The identified 4 miRNA group can aid in differentiation of MPM from RMPs

Biomarker	Reference	n	Groups	Method	Findings	Conclusion
	Tomasetti et al,[143] 2012	45/121	NSCLC, healthy	Serum real-time qPCR	miR-126-3p was able to distinguish patients with MPM from healthy controls (AUC, 0.894) and NSCLC (AUC, 0.751)	miR-126-3p can serve as a diagnostic (and prognostic) biomarker for MPM
	Busacca et al,[139] 2010	24/24	—	Tissue; miRNA microarray analysis; real-time qPCR	Analysis of MPM specimen revealed overexpression of miR-17-5p, miR-21, miR-29a, miR-30c, miR-30e-5p, miR-106a, and miR-143. Certain miRNA correlate with specific pathologic subtypes	The identified miRNA points can be helpful diagnostic and prognostic biomarkers
	Guled et al,[140] 2009	17/17	—	Tissue; miRNA microarray analysis	miRNA microarray analysis of MPM revealed overexpression of miR-30b, miR-32, miR-483-3p, miR-584, and miR-885-3p and downregulation of miR-9, miR-7-1, and miR-203	Certain combination of miRNA points can serve as diagnostic biomarkers for MPM
DNA methylation	Guarrera et al,[170] 2019	163/300	Cancer-free asbestos exposed	Blood; genome-wide methylation array technique	The identified set of methylation markers was able to distinguish MPM AUC, 0.81–0.89	Blood DNA methylation array can serve as a complementary tool in screening high-risk group for MPM
HMGB1	Ying et al,[182] 2017	15/497	Healthy, asbestos exposed <10 y, asbestos exposed >10 y, pleural plaques, diagnosed with asbestosis	Serum, ELISA	HMBG1 was able to differentiate MPM from all other groups (except for asbestosis) with high sensitivity and specificity AUC for differentiating MPM from healthy, 0.94	HMBG1 is a potential biomarker for diagnosis of MPM in asbestos-exposed population
	Napolitano et al,[183] 2016	22/100	Asbestos exposed, benign effusion, other malignant effusion, healthy	Serum	Fibulin-3 was able to distinguish MPM with high accuracy AUC, 0.959 Combining fibulin-3 with HMGB1 resulted in higher sensitivity, and specificity for differentiating MPM	Combined panel of fibulin-3 and HMGB1, is effective in diagnosing MPM
Calretinin		34/170	Healthy	Plasma, ELISA		

(continued on next page)

Table 1
(continued)

Biomarker	Author, Year	N (MPM/Total)	Compared Groups	Method	Results	Conclusion
	Johnen et al,[199] 2018				Calretinin was able to distinguish MPM from controls AUC, 0.74 Combining calretinin and mesothelin resulted in higher performance AUC, 0.83	Calretinin is highly specific but not very sensitive for MPM. Calretinin-mesothelin combined panel can provide a test with high performance in diagnosis of MPM
	Johnen et al,[196] 2017	199/434	Healthy	Serum/plasma, ELISA	Calretinin was able to differentiate MPM from controls with high sensitivity and specificity AUC, 0.87–0.95 depending on the county of origin	Calretinin can serve as a biomarker for diagnosis of MPM along with other markers
	Raiko et al,[195] 2010	42/174	Asbestos exposed, healthy	Plasma, ELISA	Calretinin was significantly higher in MPM compared with asbestos exposed and healthy (no AUC provided)	Calretinin has high sensitivity in diagnosis of MPM and can be used a biomarker for diagnosis of MPM
TRX	Demir et al,[98] 2016	42/131	Asbestos exposed, healthy	Serum (various markers, including TRX, SMRP, EGFR, mesothelin, syndecan-1, fibulin-3)	TRX (and SMRP) showed graded increase: control-asbestos-MPM, and was able to distinguish MPM from other groups AUC, 0.72	TRX and SMRP provide better diagnostic accuracy than EGFR, mesothelin, syndecan-1, fibulin-3

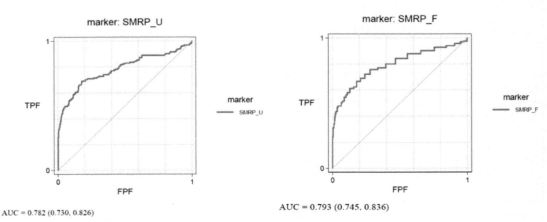

ROC curve for UCLA's measurement of SMRP   ROC curve for Fujirebio's measurement of SMRP

AUC = 0.782 (0.730, 0.826)   AUC = 0.793 (0.745, 0.836)

Fig. 1. EDRN validation trial results for SMRP as an MPM biomarker.

0.720 (95% CI, 0.562–0.853) with statistical significance, revealing evidence that SMRP can be increased within a year before diagnosis (**Fig. 2**). Analysis of data at 1- to 2-year intervals, however, did not show a statistically significant AUC, most likely due to small case number. Other studies similarly show an increase in SMRP levels in the year before diagnosis, but SMRP levels lack adequate sensitivity to serve as a reliable standalone screening test, and current evidence collectively suggests that it lacks sufficient sensitivity to be used for screening in high-risk population.[50–52]

SMRP has been found to be valuable in monitoring therapy. In a study of 28 patients with MPM undergoing therapy with copper reducing agent tetrathiomolybdate,[53] MESOMARK assays were used to measure serum SMRP levels during the therapeutic period and over the progression time. SMRP levels significantly decreased immediately after surgery. Interestingly, a gradual increase over time was seen in 82% of patients with progressive disease, whereas such increases were not observed in 45.5% of patients with stable disease, the difference of which was statistically

significant. Utility of SMRP in monitoring therapy was subsequently validated by other studies.[54–58] Schneider and colleagues[59] found that, at a cutoff value of 1.35 nmol/L, SMRP levels inversely correlated with OS. Nonetheless, prognostic value of SMRP on OS was lost in multivariate analysis limited to epithelial MPM. Conversely, Burt and colleagues[54] showed that, in patients with epithelial histology, serum SMRP level significantly decreased immediately after macroscopic complete resection, and preoperative SMRP levels were independently associated with poor disease-free survival. Specifically, the study showed that percentage change in serial postoperative SMRP values at cutoff at 48% was able to predict disease recurrence with 90% sensitivity and 93% specificity. Three prospective studies with a total of 304 patients with MPM, also showed that high baseline SMRP levels were significantly associated with shorter survival.[59–61] In addition, Creaney and colleagues[57] showed that postchemotherapy decrease in SMRP strongly correlated with longer survival. A meta-analysis of 8 studies with 579 patients with MPM showed that serum

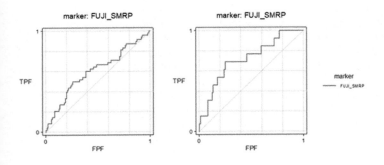

marker: FUJI_SMRP   marker: FUJI_SMRP

Fig. 2. ROC curve for SMRP, all cases, AUC = 0.604 (95% CI, 0.489, 0.699); ROC curve for SMRP, cases less than 1 year before diagnosis, AUC = 0.720 (95% CI, 0.562, 0.853).

SMRP level significantly correlated with survival.[62] Overall, current evidence suggest good prognostic value for SMRP.

Currently, the prognostic role of MSLN in MPM is inconclusive. Several studies showed no association between serum MSLN level and progression-free survival or OS.[52,63,64] On the other hand a prospective study of 41 patients with MPM showed that a 10% increase in serum MSLN was able to predict radiographic progression with 96% sensitivity. In addition, a rising MSLN level at 6 months was associated with significantly worse OS compared with stable or falling levels (175 versus 448 days, respectively).[65] A systematic review of 8 studies showed that serum MSLN levels correlated with radiographic progression and survival.[66]

MPF has not been studied in as much detail as the other mesothelin-related markers. Previous studies showed that serum MPF levels were significantly higher in patients with MPM compared with patients with benign asbestos-related diseases, lung cancer, or healthy individuals.[67,68] Current evidence suggests that MPF and SMRPs have comparable diagnostic performance in differentiating MPM from other diseases.[40,69] Nonetheless, a key limitation in using SMRPs and MPF for diagnosis of MPM is that their levels can significantly be affected by many physiologic and/or pathologic factors, including age, renal function, and body mass index (BMI).[55,63,70,71]

Osteopontin

Osteopontin (OPN) is a glycoprotein secreted into the extracellular matrix that has major roles in several physiologic processes, including cell-matrix interaction, cell migration via integrin and CD44 receptors, immunologic regulation, as well as tumor development.[72–76] Increased serum OPN levels are seen in various cancers, such as colon, breast, and lung cancer, and in MPM.[77–82]

Both in vitro asbestos-exposed cells and in vivo rat models for asbestos-induced carcinogenesis, exhibited upregulation of OPN.[83] Pass and colleagues[80] were the first to discover and describe the potential role of OPN in MPM pathogenesis, using HG1 Affymetrix array to detect a 9-fold increase in OPN RNA expression in 48 MPMs compared with matched normal peritoneum as a normal mesothelial control. The early study used a commercially available OPN ELISA and found serum OPN levels to be significantly higher in patients with MPM compared with asbestos-exposed and asbestos-unexposed individuals, although the last 2 were not significantly different. Furthermore, OPN showed high accuracy in differentiating stage I patients with MPM from asbestos-exposed individuals, but it was not able to distinguish MPM from other asbestos exposure-related pathologies.[61] Despite initial promising results, due to low specificity and conflicting results of later studies, utility of OPN in early diagnosis of MPM became contentious.[61,84–87] Two studies showed that OPN had higher diagnostic performance when measured in serum compared with plasma, likely due to higher stability in the serum.[84,88] A meta-analysis of 6 studies with 360 patients with MPM and 546 non-MPM controls found a pooled sensitivity of 65% and specificity of 81% for OPN, with an AUC of ROC of 0.83.[89]

Although collective data support the utility of OPN as an adjunctive biomarker in diagnosis of MPM, its prognostic role might be more prominent. Cappia and colleagues[90] investigated the expression of OPN in short-term and long-term survivors of MPM and found that, at a cutoff value of 145 histologic scoring (HScore), OPN was an independent prognostic predictor for MPM. Furthermore, other studies showed independent association of low baseline plasma OPN levels with favorable progression-free survival and OS in patients with MPM.[52,61] Grigoriu and colleagues[61] found serum OPN and serum MSLN to be independent prognostic factors in MPM. In addition, Hollevoet and colleagues[52] conducted a study on 45 patients with MPM during and after chemotherapy, and compared OPN levels in patients with stable disease, partial response, and progressive disease. Multivariate analysis confirmed an association of unfavorable prognosis with increased OPN. The landmark study by Pass and colleagues[91] was an international blinded study with a discovery set of 83 MPMs from the US and a validation set of 111 MPMs from Canada that expanded prognostic accuracy of MPM by using OPN and MSLN as biomarkers. In both sets, there were individual associations between higher levels of OPN and MSLN and worse prognosis. Consequently, plasma OPN or MSLN were incorporated into a baseline predictive prognostic index model, resulting in substantially and statistically significant improvement in Harrell's C-statistic. The final combined model consisting of log-OPN, the EORTC clinical prognostic index, and hemoglobin was an independently significant predictor of survival. Furthermore, the combined biomarker and clinical model significantly improved Harrell's C-index from the clinical model, from 0.718 (0.67–0.77) to 0.801 (0.77–0.84). Of note, recent studies showed a prognostic value for OPN in malignant peritoneal mesothelioma.[92] Bonotti and colleagues[93] performed consecutive measurements of OPN, SMRP, and vimentin during follow-up of 56 patients with MPM and assessed their response to therapy. They found that percentage differences between 2 consecutive measurements of each of those biomarkers, significantly correlated with the clinical course, specifically disease category: stable disease, partial response, and disease progression.

Fibulin-3

Fibulin-3 (FBLN3) is a glycoprotein encoded by the epidermal growth factor (EGF)-containing fibulin-like extracellular matrix protein-1 (EFEMP-1) gene and belongs to a family of extracellular proteins expressed in the basement membranes of blood vessels. It is involved in cell growth, adhesion, motility, and particularly tumorigenesis.[94,95] An early study using an HG1 Affymetrix array showed a 7-fold increase in EFEMP1 RNA expression ($P = 10^{-9}$) in 48 MPMs compared with matched normal peritoneum.[96] Tert-transformed mesothelial cell transfection with EFEMP1 exhibits increased proliferation, colony formation, and migration, whereas siRNA FBLN3 transfection into 2 MPM cell lines reveals the opposite functional characteristics (Pass H,unpublished data, 2017). Using the only available ELISA in 2012 (Cloud Clone, China), Pass and colleagues[96] found FBLN3 levels capable of differentiating patients with MPM from healthy asbestos-exposed controls and those affected by other types of cancers. In the study set, a plasma FBLN3 level cutoff of 52.8 ng/mL exhibited 96.7% sensitivity and 95.5% specificity in differentiating patients with and without MPM. Although the blinded validation cohort from the Princess Margaret Cancer Center corroborated earlier results, the level of accuracy was slightly lower.[96] In addition, they found that PE FBLN3 level could discriminate patients with MPM from those with PEs unrelated to MPM. Moreover, the pleural effusion FBLN3 level had prognostic value, with patients having high levels surviving shorter times than those with low levels.[96] Agha and colleagues[97] compared serum and PE FBLN3 levels in 25 patients with MPM, 11 patients with metastatic pleural carcinoma (Mets) and 9 patients with benign PEs and observed similar results to those of Pass and colleagues[96]: serum and PE FBLN3 levels were significantly higher in patients with MPM compared with those with metastatic effusion of carcinoma or benign pleural effusion. At cutoff points of 150 and 66.5 ng/mL, PE and serum FBLN3 levels successfully discriminated between patients with MPM and patients with Mets, respectively (PE AUC, 0.878; serum AUC, 0.776).

Moreover, PE and serum FBLN3 levels were capable of distinguishing patients with MPM from those with benign PEs at cutoff points of 127.5 and 18 ng/mL, respectively (PE AUC, 0.909; serum AUC, 0.931).[97] In a later study, including 42 patients with MPM, serum FBLN3 levels were significantly higher in patients with MPM compared with asbestos-exposed individuals and healthy controls.[98] Jiang and colleagues[99] also explored the diagnostic role of FBLN3 in MPM, and reported that serum FBLN3 was able to distinguish patients with MPM from healthy controls, asbestos-exposed individuals, patients with pleural plaques, and patients with asbestosis with AUCs of 0.92, 0.88, 0.90, and 0.81, respectively.

Nonetheless, the role of FBLN3 as a biomarker has been controversial since later studies had conflicting results. The comparative study by Kaya and colleagues[100] of 43 patients with MPM and 40 healthy controls revealed a significantly higher serum FBLN3 in patients with MPM and, at the best cutoff point of 36.6 ng/mL, FBLN3 had 93.0% sensitivity and 90.0% specificity for diagnosis of MPM (AUC, 0.976). It is of interest that studies that did not find diagnostic power of FBLN3 in the plasma indeed validated the prognostic value for PE FBLN3 in MPM. Kirschner and colleagues[101] investigated serum and PE FBLN3 levels in 2 different series and reported plasma FBLN3 to be significantly higher in patients with MPM in only 1 series. Diagnostic accuracy was found to be low for plasma FBLN3. On the other hand, although PE FBLN3 levels in patients with MPM and controls were not significantly different, lower levels of PE FBLN3 correlated with significantly improved survival in patients with MPM, and were independently associated with prognosis with a hazard ratio of 9.92. Creaney and colleagues[64] performed a study of 82 patients with MPM and similarly found PE FBLN3 level to be a significant prognostic predictor in patients with MPM. However, their study indicated low sensitivity for both serum and PE FBLN3 levels, inferior to that of MSLN. Furthermore, in a later study, including 33 patients with MPM, PE FBLN3 level could not distinguish patients with MPM from those with other pathologies.[102]

A meta-analysis of studies using serum FBLN3 for diagnosis of MPM included 7 studies with a total of 468 MPM and revealed a pooled sensitivity of 62% (95% CI, 45%–77%) and a specificity of 82% (95% CI, 73%–89%) (AUC of ROC, 0.81).[103]

Due to inconsistencies observed with the sole use of FBLN3 USCN ELISA, further investigations were initiated by the National Cancer Institute's

Early Detection Research Network Mesothelioma Biomarker Discovery Laboratory (EDRN MPM BDL) for the development of alternative assays. Consequently, a custom MRM mass spectroscopy assay for FBLN3 was reported to distinguish 15 MPMs from 15 asbestos-exposed controls, revealing markedly better AUC of 0.82 compared with earlier results observed by Australian investigators (AUC, 0.69) using the USCN ELISA. This was further supported by later studies using newer FBLN3 ELISAs, including the LS-Biosciences Chemoluminscent human EFEMP1 ELISA, to compare MPM and asbestos-exposed serum FBLN3 levels that reported an AUC of 0.93 (Pass H, personal communication, IASLC Targeted Meeting, 2020). Another significant contribution by MPM BDL was development of a unique Slow Off-Rate Modified Aptamer (SOMAmer) Luminex assay using a FBLN3 SOMAmer that revealed an AUC of 0.98. In addition, the SOMAmer assay was able to differentiate plasma obtained from patients with MPM PE, from those with non-MPM PE, with a remarkable AUC of 0.93. More recently, using a novel FBLN 3 monoclonal antibody, mAB382, a novel sandwich ELISA has been constructed in the MPM BDL, in collaboration with researchers who first described EFEMP1 expression in glioblastoma,[104] and has yielded promising results. Results from currently ongoing blinded validations of FBLN3 with other MPM and asbestos-exposed cohorts are pending.

Proteomics (Multiplex Protein Signature) and Glycomics

The proteome is defined as the complete set of proteins produced in an organism, system, or biological context, at a certain time, under specific circumstances. Proteomics has resulted in identification of various useful protein signatures that can assist in diagnosis and management of different malignancies, including MPM.[105–107] Somalogic, Boulder, Colorado, developed a remarkable proteomic platform for MPM, using over 1100 SOMAmers. SOMAmers are short, single-stranded deoxynucleotides designed to attach to specific protein targets. They are modified to be selectively eluted from the protein during steps to concentrate and quantitate the proteins that they bind.[108,109] One unique feature of SOMAmers is that multiplexing them allows for quantification of many proteins with very small amounts of sample. In a multicenter case-control study of 117 patients with MPM and 142 asbestos-exposed controls, SOMAmers were used to screen more than 1000 proteins, identified 64 candidate biomarkers, and created a 13-

marker random forest classifier that was able to differentiate patients with MPM from asbestos-exposed controls with both sensitivity and specificity of greater than 90% (AUC, 0.99), revealing superior performance to MSLN.[107] Importantly, the 13 SOMAmer panel was later validated in 2 other cohorts.

More recently, White and colleagues[110] performed a study using quantitative mass spectrometry to explore MPM proteomic profile. They identified an explicit group of upregulated proteins in MPM effusions, capable of distinguishing MPM PE from benign reactive and adenocarcinoma-associated PEs.

Glycomics is a technique that allows for quantification of serum glycosylated moieties. Although earlier research had promising results, later studies were unable to validate the previously identified signatures for diagnosis and prognosis of MPM.[111] Therefore, further research is required to elucidate the role of glycomics in MPM.[110,112]

Genomics and Epigenomics

Some of the first attempts for genomic modeling of mesothelioma involved transcriptomic prognostication. Using a study and validation set, Pass and colleagues[113] identified a 27-gene classifier for patients with MPM that was able to predict time to progression and survival after cytoreduction and postoperative adjuvant therapy.[114] Brigham and Women's Hospital has focused on detection and validation of microRNA (miRNA) ratios for MPM prognostication.[114–117] In a recent study, Zhou and colleagues[118] developed and validated a 3-gene prognostic signature for MPM that was able to classify patients with MPM into low- and high-risk patients with significantly different OS. In an early study, representative oligonucleotide microarray analysis was used to quantify copy-number abnormalities (CNA) in patients with MPM who presented with recurrence at variable intervals after surgery.[119] Patients with early recurrence were found to have significantly greater increase in CNA and frequent deletions in chromosomes 22q12.2, 19q13.32, and 17p13.1 (55%–74%). These data suggested a prognostic role for CNA in MPM. More complex techniques, such as next-generation sequencing (NGS) moved the biomarker discovery in MPM to new levels. Whole-exome sequencing of pleural MPM in collaboration with the Broad Institute, resulted in identification of 517 somatic mutations across 490 mutated genes.[19] The most frequent genetic alterations included BAP1, NF2, CDKN2A, and CUL1. These findings were subsequently

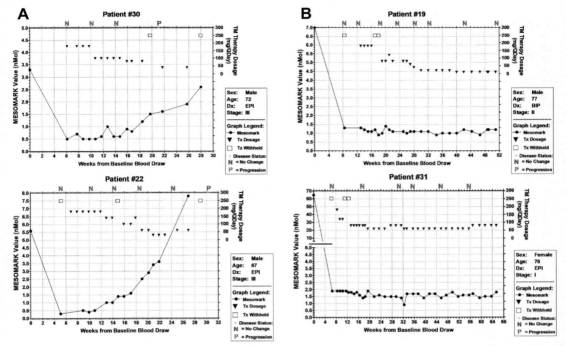

Fig. 3. Examples of patients with recurring disease (*A*) and with stable disease (*B*); patients diagnosed with mesothelioma were monitored using MESOMARK during the course of chemotherapy. Serum concentrations of mesothelin were measured before surgery and during the course of treatment postsurgery.

validated and expanded by larger studies from Brigham and Women's[120] and The Cancer Genome Atlas (TCGA).[121] BAP1 has emerged as the gene with the highest number of derangements in MPM, with diagnostic and prognostic implications. Studies from Bott and colleagues[17] were seminal in the discovery of mutated BAP1 in MPM, and Testa and colleagues[122] and Carbone and colleagues[123] were the first to describe germ line alterations of the gene and the association of these germ line mutations with familial mesothelioma. Shinozaki and colleagues[21] found that BAP1 loss and high EZH2 expression were highly specific in differentiating MPM from benign mesothelial proliferations, and that combination of both biomarkers improved diagnostic accuracy to a sensitivity of 90% and specificity of 100%. Moreover, Carbone and colleagues reported that germline mutations of BAP1 were associated with longer than expected survival,[18,124] and this has been validated in at least 1 other study.[125]

Few other studies found homozygous deletion of CDKN2A to be a prognostic factor in MPM.[121,126,127] These results corroborated with earlier findings of Chou and colleagues[128] that BAP1-negative and p16-positive (CDKN2A-positive) phenotype was associated with significantly longer survival.

Tissue and Circulating MicroRNAs

miRNAs are small noncoding RNAs involved in RNA silencing and posttranscriptional regulation of gene expression, and they have a key role in regulating various cellular processes, such as proliferation, differentiation, apoptosis, angiogenesis, and invasion.[129–133] Specific signatures of miRNAs are exhibited by tumor cells, either secreted actively or released passively after cell death.[134,135] MPM miRNA expression profiles have been extensively explored over the past few years.[136–148] An early tissue-based study found that mir-29c* was an independent predictor of survival, along with stage and lymph node involvement, regardless of histology. Data suggested mir-29c* to be an independent prognostic marker for predicting time to progression and OS after surgery, and increased miR-29c* expression was associated with significantly higher survival.[141] Furthermore, the mechanism of mir-29c* was found to be through epigenetic regulation of the tumor via downregulation of DNA methyltransferases, along with upregulation of demethylating genes. Subsequently, the prognostic role of mir-29c* in MPM was validated by TCGA (**Figs. 3** and **4**) (Gordon Robertson, personal communication, 2015).

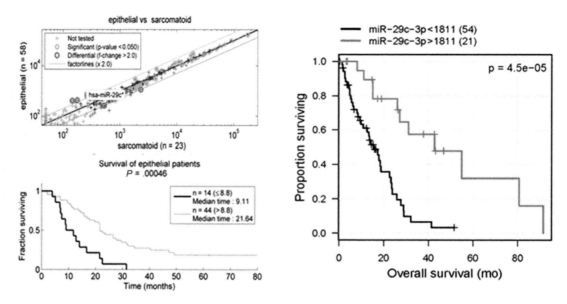

Fig. 4. mir 29c* and MPM. Left panel: significant increase of the mir in epithelial mesothelioma and loss of the mir associated with poor prognosis. Right panel: validation in 75 TCGA patients with MPM.

Although various studies have attempted to elucidate the diagnostic and prognostic role of miRNAs in MPM, there has been minimal overlap in findings of different studies and most models lack validation. The observed discrepancies may partially be explained by differences in normalizers/housekeepers. Two previous studies reported overexpression of miR-30b, miR-32, miR-483-3p, miR-584, miR-885-3p, miR-17-5p, miR-21, miR-29a, miR-30c, miR-30e-5p, miR-106a, and miR-143, and downregulation of miR-9, miR-7-1, and miR-203 in MPM.[139,140] Interestingly, correlation between certain miRNAs and specific histologic subtypes was observed in both studies. Loss of miR-31 (associated with homozygous loss of 9p21.3 chromosome in MPM) has correlated with tumor suppressor activity.[142,143] Although an early study found miR-126-3p capable of discriminating patients with MPM from healthy controls,[143] a later study provided conflicting results and found it unable to distinguish between patients with MPM and asbestos-exposed controls.[147] In the study by Matboli and colleagues[149] of 60 patients with MPM, miR-548a-3p and miR-20a sera levels could individually distinguish patients with MPM from 20 asbestos-exposed and 20 healthy controls with high sensitivity. A combined panel of both biomarkers resulted in sensitivity of 100%.

Most recently, the novel platform HTG EdgeSeq miRNA whole transcriptome assay was used to measure expression of 2083 human miRNA transcripts. When combined with NGS, this platform uses only 15 μL of serum or plasma. Preliminary results were promising, showing that a 7-serum miRNA signature was able to differentiate 93 MPMs from 53 asbestos-exposed pipe fitters with an AUC of 0.953.[150]

Further upregulated miRNAs reported in MPM are miRNA 197-3p, miRNA-1281, miRNA 32-3p,[151,152] miR-625-3p,[138] miR-103a-3p,[137,153] miR-30e-3p,[152] and miR-2053.[154]

One study found that expression of miR-17-5p and miR-30c correlated with survival in sarcomatoid MPM.[139] In addition, upregulation of miR-31 was associated with the presence of a sarcomatoid component and worse prognosis in patients with that histologic subtype.[155] Fassina and colleagues[156] found that tissue levels of miR-205 were lower in biphasic and sarcomatoid MPM histologic subtypes and higher in epithelioid type.

Kirschner and colleagues[157] performed a study on patients undergoing extrapleural pneumonectomy (EPP) or palliative surgery (P/D) to investigate the association between miRNA expression and OS. They developed a miR-Score consisting of a 6-miRNA signature (miR-21-5p, miR-23a-3p, miR-30e-5p, miR-221-3p, miR-222-3p, and miR-31-5p), which was able to predict long survival in patients undergoing EPP and P/D with 92.3% and 71.9% accuracy, respectively. In addition, Lamberti and colleagues[136] found 2 distinct serum miRNA signatures with diagnostic and prognostic significance in patients with MPM. Consequent to earlier findings, miR-29c*, miR-92a, and miR-625-

3p were validated as encouraging diagnostic markers for MPM.[138,141] In a strong validation test, De Santi and colleagues[158] reported significant differential expression of miR-185, miR-197, and miR-299 in patients with MPM and identified a 2-miRNA prognostic signature, consisting of Let-7c-5p and miR-151a-5p. Andersen and colleagues[159] performed a comparative analysis of MPM tumor tissues and nonneoplastic control specimen and found that DNA-hypermethylation downregulated miR-126 and its host gene EGFL7 and resulted in lower survival in patients with MPM.

Other studies found high tissue levels of miR-137,[160] miR-1, miR-335-5p, and miR-566 associated with a poor prognosis, whereas high tissue expression of miR-16, miR-486, miR-146a-5p, miR-378a-3p, miR-451a, and miR-1246 correlated with better outcome.[161] A study of 60 patients with MPM revealed hsa-miR-2053 to be an independent prognostic factor for MPM.[154]

Circulating Tumor DNA

Circulating tumor DNA (ctDNA) is defined as the portion of circulating cell-free DNA (cfDNA) that is released into the blood either through active secretion, or via tumor apoptosis and necrosis.[162,163] cfDNAs containing tumor mutations are detected at higher concentrations in patients with cancer and contain mutations present in the tumor.[164] Contrary to other malignancies, studies on ctDNA in MPM are limited. Although data support the feasibility of the technique, sensitivity is reported to be low. Whole-exome sequencing with validation of the tumor-specific variants by digital droplet PCR was performed in 10 patients with MPM and detection of patient-specific, selected variants was observed only in 3 treatment-naive patients with MPM, either in one or both independent droplet digital PCR runs.[165] Based on earlier findings that miR-34b/c is downregulated in 90% of MPMs, a Japanese group specifically investigated the degree of miR-34b/c methylation in serum-circulating DNA using a digital methylation-specific PCR (MSP) assay.[166] They used a technique utilizing digital droplet PCR methods in combination with MSP, originally evolved from MSP.[167] The reported sensitivity in the discovery and validation sets were 76.9% and 59.1%, and specificities were 90% and 100%, respectively. Further improvement of accuracy was observed with advancing stages of disease.

DNA Methylation

DNA methylation is an epigenetic modification occurring at specific regulatory regions of genes. Methylation patterns can be affected by several factors, including environmental exposure, aging, and various types of disease and therapy.[168] DNA methylation profile has been shown to successfully distinguish MPM cells from normal pleural cells.[169] Furthermore, the DNA methylation profile in peripheral blood, in isolation or combined with other biomarkers, might be helpful in the diagnosis of MPM.[144,170] In one study with a discovery test and a test set of MPMs and asbestos-exposed controls, a genome-wide methylation array was used to identify novel DNA methylation markers from whole blood. Aiming the top differentially methylated signals, 7 single cytosine-guanine dinucleotides and 5 genomic regions of coordinated methylation were identified in both cohorts. Subsequently, a model was created using cytosine-guanine dinucleotides (CpG) methylation levels, along with clinical characteristics of age, sex, and asbestos exposure levels, and revealed an AUC of 0.89.[170] Change in the methylation profiles over time in at-risk asbestos-exposed populations is currently unknown and yet to be explored.

Circulating Tumor Cells

Circulating tumor cells (CTCs) are cells that have detached from a primary tumor or a metastatic site and are circulating in the bloodstream. They become more abundant as cancer develops toward more advanced stages. In contrast to other cancers where methods of counting CTCs have been found helpful for diagnosis, in MPM these methods have limited utility due to low sensitivity.[171–173] Recently, however, CTC capture with microfluidics has improved the efficacy of CTC quantitation in MPM. The CTC-Chip is a novel microfluidic device developed by Chikaishi and colleagues,[174] in which the capture antibody was one against podoplanin, which is abundantly expressed on MPM. The CTC-Chip was found to have higher diagnostic value for MPM. Earlier stages of disease showed that lower numbers of cells and CTCs were positive in only 68% of clinical samples. Highest accuracy was seen in comparison of CTCs in earlier stages to those with stages IIIB and IV (AUC, 0.851). In addition, CTC count $\geq$2 cells/mL was associated with significantly worse prognosis ($P = .030$).

INFLAMMATORY AND ANGIOGENIC FACTORS
High-Mobility Group Box 1

High-mobility group box 1 (HMGB1) is among the most important chromatin proteins that interacts with nucleosomes and transcription factors and facilitates binding of DNA to other proteins. Accordingly, it regulates transcription, DNA repair, proliferation, and inflammation.[175,176] Recognized as a damage-associated molecular pattern, HMGB1 is released by cells undergoing necrosis in physiologic states. Conversely, in pathologic states a hyperacetylated form of HMGB1 can be secreted by inflammatory and cancer cells.[177–179] Exposure of human mesothelial cells to asbestos provokes programmed necrosis and results in the release of HMGB1, along with activation of Nalp3 inflammasome, and eventually cell alteration.[12,15,16,180,181] In a study of 15 patients with MPM, serum HMGB1 level was significantly higher in patients with MPM compared with non-MPM asbestos-exposed individuals.[182] In another study, total blood HMGB1 levels were found to be higher in patients with MPM and asbestos-exposed individuals compared with healthy controls. More importantly, hyperacetylated HMGB1 was significantly higher in patients with MPM compared with asbestos-exposed and healthy controls.[183] Validation of these findings is forthcoming. Combined use of HMGB1 and FBLN3 resulted in improved accuracy. One study showed that, at a cutoff value of 9 ng/mL, there was a significant negative correlation between serum HMGB1 level and survival, suggesting a potential prognostic role for HMGB1.[86] Furthermore, in a systematic review and meta-analysis by Wu and colleagues[184] of 18 studies on HMGB1 overexpression in various types of cancer, HMGB1 was found to be a prognostic marker for MPM.

Peripheral Blood-Based Markers

Given the well-established role of chronic inflammation in pathophysiology of various cancers, including MPM, many studies have investigated the role of inflammation-based scores, such as lymphocyte-to-monocyte ratio (LMR), neutrophil-to-lymphocyte ratio (NLR), and platelet-to-lymphocyte ratio in diagnosis and prognosis of MPM. A retrospective study of 150 patients with MPM found increased LMR significantly associated with prolonged OS. Specifically, median OS was 14 months in patients with LMR ≥ 2.74 compared with 5 months in patients with LMR less than 2.74. Multivariate analysis confirmed LMR to be an independent prognostic marker for OS in MPM.[185] Conversely, the prognostic role of NLR is somewhat controversial. Although many studies consistently found baseline NLR to be an independent predictor of improved survival,[186–189] other studies failed to show similar results.[190,191]

A study of 55 patients with MPM showed that late-stage patients with MPM had significantly

higher plasma circulating complement component 4d (C4d) levels compared with early-stage patients, and that high circulating C4d levels correlated with higher tumor volume. Furthermore, after induction chemotherapy, plasma C4d levels were significantly higher in patients with stable and progressive disease compared with those with partial or major response. In multivariate analysis, patients with low C4d levels at diagnosis were found to have significantly better OS.[192]

Calretinin

Calretinin is a vitamin D-dependent calcium-binding protein similar to S-100 and is a member of EF-hand protein family. Encoded by the CALB2 gene, calretinin was first detected in neurons and later on mesothelial cell surfaces and has been found to be overexpressed in MPM.[193,194] A calretinin assay developed by Raiko and colleagues[195] could differentiate patients with MPM from asbestos-exposed and healthy controls. In addition, the assay was able to distinguish asbestos-exposed individuals from healthy controls. Later studies showed corroborative results. In comparing MPM and controls, calretinin had sensitivity of 71% for a predefined specificity of 95%, with AUC ranging between 0.77 and 0.95 depending on the gender and the country of origin of the specimen.[196–198] Furthermore, blood calretinin levels could prediagnose mesothelioma 1 to 15 months before definitive diagnosis in an asbestos-exposed population with an AUC of 0.77.[199] Additional use of serum MSLN enhanced the accuracy to AUC of 0.85. In another study, calretinin expression was found to be an independent predictor of survival in patients with MPM.[200] Following earlier promising results, validation studies for calretinin and FBLN3 are currently underway.

ENOX2

ENOX2 (Ecto-NOX disulfide-thiol exchanger 2) is a cell surface protein, a member of the NOX family of NADPH oxidases that is involved in oxidization of reduced pyridine nucleotides and is essential for cell growth.[201] Specific cancer cells exhibit tissue-specific patterns of ENOX2 transcript variants.[202] ENOX2 proteins are released in circulation and can be detected at an early stage in particular cancers, including breast, lung, colon, prostate, and ovarian cancer.[202] Specific ENOX2 protein transcript variants characteristic of MPM were identified by Morré and colleagues[203] that could be detected in sera of patients 4 to 10 years before developing clinical symptoms.

Thioredoxin-1

Thioredoxin-1 (TRX) is a conserved antioxidant protein, well known for its regulatory disulfide reductase activity, and has a critical role in decreasing ROS levels.[204] Overexpression of TRX has been detected in patients with MPM.[15] In a study by Demir and colleagues,[98] TRX and SMRP exhibited a graded increase among controls, asbestos-exposed individuals, and patients with MPM, respectively. TRX showed a sensitivity of 92.9% and specificity of 77.6% in diagnosis of MPM.

Vascular Endothelial Growth Factor

Vascular endothelial growth factor (VEGF) is a signal protein and a key stimulator of neoangiogenesis and has been found to be overexpressed in many malignant tissues, including MPM.[205–207] VEGF levels in PE were significantly higher in patients with MPM compared with those with PEs related to nonmalignant pleural diseases or lung cancer.[208] Hirayama and colleagues[208] determined 2000 pg/mL to be the optimal cutoff value between low and high VEGF-A levels in MPM PE, showing a significant correlation with survival. The median survival was 12 and 4 months in the low- and high-level groups, respectively.[208] Similarly, higher levels of serum VEGF were found in patients with MPM compared with those with nonmalignant asbestos-related diseases.[209] At a cutoff at 460 pg/mL, there was a strong correlation between high serum VEGF level and shorter survival. Another study showed that VEGF staining correlates with short survival, tumor stage, and prognosis in MPM.[207] Nowak and colleagues[210] found that, in patients with MPM treated with multitarget tyrosine kinase inhibitor sunitinib malate, baseline serum levels of VEGF-A and VEGF receptor 2 (VEGFR-2) correlated with radiological response.

Miscellaneous Potential Biomarkers

Stockhammer and colleagues[211] found strong prognostic value for PE transforming growth factor β (TGF-β) levels in patients with MPM. Subgroup analysis showed that PE TGF-β levels were highly prognostic in epithelioid histology, but there was only a trend in the nonepithelioid group.[211] Conversely, the study showed no diagnostic and prognostic power for circulating TGF-β levels in patients with MPM. In addition, there was no correlation between PE and circulating TGF-β levels.

Serum matrix metalloproteinase 9 (MMP-9) is an extracellular protein that has a role in various physiologic and pathologic processes, including development, wound healing, cell migration, and metastasis.[212] One study showed that MMP-9 overexpression in correlation with MSLN overexpression was associated with increased tumor invasion and decreased survival in patients with MPM.[41] Štrbac and colleagues[213,214] identified certain MMP-9 genotypes that were associated with significantly shorter OS and time to progression compared with other alleles. A later study showed that although serum MMP9 concentration was different in patients with complete versus partial response and in patients with stable versus progressive disease, the concentration differences did not reach statistical significance and thus not associated with survival or treatment response.[215]

Bridging integrator 1 (BIN1) is a member of BAR domain superfamily involved in endocytosis, cell division, and migration.[216] In a study of 67 patients with MPM, Ahmadzada and colleagues[217] found high BIN1 expression to be a favorable prognostic biomarker for MPM and associated with tumor-infiltrating lymphocytes (TILs).

Metallothionein (MT) is a family of cysteine-rich low-molecular-mass proteins that have capacity of binding heavy metals through thiol groups of their cysteine residues.[218] In a retrospective study of 105 patients with MPM, both OS and progression-free survival negatively correlated with detectable MT expression, suggesting a possible resistance to platin-based chemotherapy associated with MT expression upregulation, found exclusively in progressive MPM samples.[219]

Aquaporin-1 (AQP1) is a cell membrane water channel protein found throughout the body that plays a role in transcellular water transport.[220] A study by Angelico and colleagues[221,222] showed that patients with AQP1 overexpression (defined as ≥50% of tumor cells showing membranous staining) had a significantly longer median OS compared with those with an AQP1 score of less than 50% (26.3 months compared with 8.9 months, respectively).

Marcq and colleagues[223] investigated immune cell composition of PE in patients with MPM and identified 2 factors with clinical value. Percentage of PD-L1+ podoplanin (PDPN)+ tumor cells was a significant prognostic factor for worse outcome, whereas CD4+ T cells were associated with better response to chemotherapy.

Later studies corroborated earlier results indicating that higher expression of peritumoral TILs correlated with improved OS, whereas PD-L1 expression inversely correlated with clinical outcomes.[224–226]

Combined Panels

Many studies have investigated various combination of biomarkers to achieve higher accuracy for diagnosis of MPM.[183,227] Jimenez-Ramirez and colleagues[227] used a mesothelin-calretinin-MPF combination and were able to obtain sensitivity of 82% in men (AUC, 0.944), and 87% in women (AUC, 0.937). In a unique study, Bonotti and colleagues[228] assessed various combinations of biomarkers in MPM and identified the 2 best 3-marker combinations as IL6-OPN-SMRP (AUC, 0.945) and IL6-OPN-Desmin (AUC, 0.950). In addition, they found the best 4-marker combination to be SMRP-OPN-IL6-Vimentin (AUC, 0.962).

In a recent study, Doi and colleagues[229] developed a novel prognostic risk classification system for MPM. Significant independent predictors of poor survival were an NLR of ≥ 5.0, along with non-epithelioid histologic type, increased serum lactate dehydrogenase levels, and a total lesion glycolysis of ≥ 525 g.

Breath analysis

Exhaled breath is composed of 2 major phases: a liquid phase containing water vapor, and a gaseous phase consisting of oxygen, carbon dioxide, nitrogen, inert gases, and a small fraction of volatile organic compounds (VOCs).[230] VOCs' origin can either be exogenous via inhalation and dermal absorption, or endogenous as a result of physiologic and pathophysiological processes, including inflammation, metabolism, and oxidative stress.[231,232] More than 3000 different VOCs have been described so far, but a single breath sample commonly contains about 200 different VOCs.[230] Because VOCs are influenced by various pathophysiological states, they have been studied as potential biomarkers for diagnosis of various benign and malignant diseases, including MPM.[30,233–235] Although gas chromatography-mass spectrometry continues to be the gold standard method for breath analysis, various other methods have been successfully used for molecular assessment of breath components, including multicapillary column ion mobility spectrometry (MCC-IMS),[236] selected ion flow tube-mass spectrometry,[237] proton transfer reaction-mass spectrometry,[187] electronic noses (eNoses), and canine scent test.[232] In a meta-analysis of various breath analysis methods, eNose and MCC-IMS were found to have the highest and the lowest accuracies, respectively (95% versus 65%).[234,238]

SUMMARY

Over the last 2 decades there have been numerous investigations on diagnostic, monitoring, and prognostic biomarkers for MPM, but thus far, only 1 biomarker has been validated as a blood-based test in North America, Europe, and Australia. The main grounds for failure of validations of other marker are scarcity of large archives of prospectively collected high-quality specimens, limited funding for performance of large-scale validation trials, and necessity of a more cohesive approach by mesothelioma investigators. The relative lack of industrial interest and support for MPM biomarker development and validation, as compared with lung cancer, is likely secondary to its smaller market and the common misconception that MPM will evade over the next few decades. There is a continued need for accurate diagnosis and early detection of the disease particularly with an increasing rate of cases secondary to familial BAP1 germline mutations and recognition of other carcinogenic fibers, such as erionite in new locations.

CLINICS CARE POINTS

- Poor prognosis of advanced staged MPM, along with cost and morbidities associated with pleural biopsy, has developed high interest in investigating biomarkers for diagnosis and monitoring of therapy in MPM.
- Studies suggest that MPM has a low mutation burden, with tumor suppressors BAP1, NF2, and CDKN2A being the most frequently mutated genes.
- Certain biomarkers have strong diagnostic values, whereas others exhibit better prognostic values.
- Combined panels have shown the most promising results in improving accuracy.
- Large coordinated validation studies are required for further assessment of practical utility of biomarkers.

DISCLOSURE

H.I. Pass reports funding from the National Cancer Institute, the Department of Defense, the Centers for Disease Control and Prevention, Genentech, and Belluck and Fox. Financial support for this article was only for H.I. Pass (5U01CA214195-04 The EDRN Mesothelioma Biomarker Discovery Laboratory). M. Carbone and H. Yang report grants from the NIH, National Cancer Institute, the US Department of Defense, and the UH Foundation through donations to support research on "Pathogenesis of Malignant Mesothelioma" from Honeywell International Inc., Riviera United-4-a Cure, and the Maurice and Joanna Sullivan Family Foundation. M. Carbone has a patent issued for

BAP1. M. Carbone and H. Yang have a patent issued for "Using Anti-HMGB1 Monoclonal Antibody or other HMGB1 Antibodies as a Novel Mesothelioma Therapeutic Strategy," and a patent issued for "HMGB1 As a Biomarker for Asbestos Exposure and Mesothelioma Early Detection." Michele Carbone is a board-certified pathologist who provides consultation for mesothelioma expertise and diagnosis. The remaining authors report no disclosures.

REFERENCES

1. Carbone M, Ly BH, Dodson RF, et al. Malignant mesothelioma: facts, myths, and hypotheses. J Cell Physiol 2012;227:44–58.
2. Baumann F, Ambrosi JP, Carbone M. Asbestos is not just asbestos: an unrecognised health hazard. Lancet Oncol 2013;14:576–8.
3. Takahashi K. Asbestos-related diseases: time for technology sharing. Occup Med (Lond) 2008;58:384–5.
4. Gazdar AF, Carbone M. Molecular pathogenesis of malignant mesothelioma and its relationship to simian virus 40. Clin Lung Cancer 2003;5:177–81.
5. Carbone M, Rizzo P, Pass H. Simian virus 40: the link with human malignant mesothelioma is well established. Anticancer Res 2000;20:875–7.
6. Carbone M. Simian virus 40 and human tumors: it is time to study mechanisms. J Cell Biochem 1999;76:189–93.
7. Kroczynska B, Cutrone R, Bocchetta M, et al. Crocidolite asbestos and SV40 are cocarcinogens in human mesothelial cells and in causing mesothelioma in hamsters. Proc Natl Acad Sci U S A 2006;103:14128–33.
8. Attanoos RL, Churg A, Galateau-Salle F, et al. Malignant mesothelioma and its non-asbestos causes. Arch Pathol Lab Med 2018;142:753–60.
9. Carbone M, Kanodia S, Chao A, et al. Consensus report of the 2015 Weinman International Conference on Mesothelioma. J Thorac Oncol 2016;11:1246–62.
10. Delgermaa V, Takahashi K, Park EK, et al. Global mesothelioma deaths reported to the World Health Organization between 1994 and 2008. Bull World Health Organ 2011;89:716–24, 724a-724c.
11. Robinson BM. Malignant pleural mesothelioma: an epidemiological perspective. Ann Cardiothorac Surg 2012;1:491–6.
12. Carbone M, Yang H. Molecular pathways: targeting mechanisms of asbestos and erionite carcinogenesis in mesothelioma. Clin Cancer Res 2012;18:598–604.
13. Bograd AJ, Suzuki K, Vertes E, et al. Immune responses and immunotherapeutic interventions in malignant pleural mesothelioma. Cancer Immunol Immunother 2011;60:1509–27.
14. Dostert C, Petrilli V, Van Bruggen R, et al. Innate immune activation through Nalp3 inflammasome sensing of asbestos and silica. Science 2008;320:674–7.
15. Qi F, Okimoto G, Jube S, et al. Continuous exposure to chrysotile asbestos can cause transformation of human mesothelial cells via HMGB1 and TNF-alpha signaling. Am J Pathol 2013;183:1654–66.
16. Yang H, Rivera Z, Jube S, et al. Programmed necrosis induced by asbestos in human mesothelial cells causes high-mobility group box 1 protein release and resultant inflammation. Proc Natl Acad Sci U S A 2010;107:12611–6.
17. Bott M, Brevet M, Taylor BS, et al. The nuclear deubiquitinase BAP1 is commonly inactivated by somatic mutations and 3p21.1 losses in malignant pleural mesothelioma. Nat Genet 2011;43:668–72.
18. Baumann F, Flores E, Napolitano A, et al. Mesothelioma patients with germline BAP1 mutations have 7-fold improved long-term survival. Carcinogenesis 2015;36:76–81.
19. Guo G, Chmielecki J, Goparaju C, et al. Whole-exome sequencing reveals frequent genetic alterations in BAP1, NF2, CDKN2A, and CUL1 in malignant pleural mesothelioma. Cancer Res 2015;75:264–9.
20. Nasu M, Emi M, Pastorino S, et al. High incidence of somatic BAP1 alterations in sporadic malignant mesothelioma. J Thorac Oncol 2015;10:565–76.
21. Shinozaki-Ushiku A, Ushiku T, Morita S, et al. Diagnostic utility of BAP1 and EZH2 expression in malignant mesothelioma. Histopathology 2017;70:722–33.
22. Kadota K, Suzuki K, Sima CS, et al. Pleomorphic epithelioid diffuse malignant pleural mesothelioma: a clinicopathological review and conceptual proposal to reclassify as biphasic or sarcomatoid mesothelioma. J Thorac Oncol 2011;6:896–904.
23. Rusch VW, Chansky K, Kindler HL, et al. The IASLC mesothelioma staging project: proposals for the M descriptors and for revision of the TNM stage groupings in the forthcoming (eighth) edition of the TNM Classification for Mesothelioma. J Thorac Oncol 2016;11:2112–9.
24. Nowak AK, Chansky K, Rice DC, et al. The IASLC mesothelioma staging project: proposals for revisions of the T descriptors in the forthcoming eighth edition of the TNM classification for pleural mesothelioma. J Thorac Oncol 2016;11:2089–99.
25. Cinausero M, Rihawi K, Cortiula F, et al. Emerging therapies in malignant pleural mesothelioma. Crit Rev Oncol Hematol 2019;144:102815.
26. Hoang CD. Surgical controversies in mesothelioma: MesoVATS addresses the role of surgical debulking. Transl Lung Cancer Res 2016;5:82–4.

27. Abdel-Rahman O. Role of postoperative radiotherapy in the management of malignant pleural mesothelioma: a propensity score matching of the SEER database. Strahlenther Onkol 2017;193:276–84.

28. Abdel-Rahman O, Elsayed Z, Mohamed H, et al. Radical multimodality therapy for malignant pleural mesothelioma. Cochrane Database Syst Rev 2018;1:Cd012605.

29. Cavallari I, Urso L, Sharova E, et al. Liquid biopsy in malignant pleural mesothelioma: state of the art, pitfalls, and perspectives. Front Oncol 2019;9:740.

30. Catino A, de Gennaro G, Di Gilio A, et al. Breath analysis: a systematic review of volatile organic compounds (VOCs) in diagnostic and therapeutic management of pleural mesothelioma. Cancers (Basel) 2019;11:831.

31. Tsim S, Stobo DB, Alexander L, et al. The diagnostic performance of routinely acquired and reported computed tomography imaging in patients presenting with suspected pleural malignancy. Lung Cancer 2017;103:38–43.

32. Tsao MS, Carbone M, Galateau-Salle F, et al. Pathologic considerations and standardization in mesothelioma clinical trials. J Thorac Oncol 2019;14:1704–17.

33. Chang K, Pastan I. Molecular cloning of mesothelin, a differentiation antigen present on mesothelium, mesotheliomas, and ovarian cancers. Proc Natl Acad Sci U S A 1996;93:136–40.

34. Hellstrom I, Raycraft J, Kanan S, et al. Mesothelin variant 1 is released from tumor cells as a diagnostic marker. Cancer Epidemiol Biomarkers Prev 2006;15:1014–20.

35. Robinson BW, Creaney J, Lake R, et al. Mesothelin-family proteins and diagnosis of mesothelioma. Lancet 2003;362:1612–6.

36. Zervos MD, Bizekis C, Pass HI. Malignant mesothelioma 2008. Curr Opin Pulm Med 2008;14:303–9.

37. Tang Z, Qian M, Ho M. The role of mesothelin in tumor progression and targeted therapy. Anticancer Agents Med Chem 2013;13:276–80.

38. Hassan R, Laszik ZG, Lerner M, et al. Mesothelin is overexpressed in pancreaticobiliary adenocarcinomas but not in normal pancreas and chronic pancreatitis. Am J Clin Pathol 2005;124:838–45.

39. Ho M, Bera TK, Willingham MC, et al. Mesothelin expression in human lung cancer. Clin Cancer Res 2007;13:1571–5.

40. Creaney J, Sneddon S, Dick IM, et al. Comparison of the diagnostic accuracy of the MSLN gene products, mesothelin and megakaryocyte potentiating factor, as biomarkers for mesothelioma in pleural effusions and serum. Dis Markers 2013;35:119–27.

41. Servais EL, Colovos C, Rodriguez L, et al. Mesothelin overexpression promotes mesothelioma cell invasion and MMP-9 secretion in an orthotopic mouse model and in epithelioid pleural mesothelioma patients. Clin Cancer Res 2012;18:2478–89.

42. Beyer HL, Geschwindt RD, Glover CL, et al. MESOMARK: a potential test for malignant pleural mesothelioma. Clin Chem 2007;53:666–72.

43. Pass HI, Wali A, Tang N, et al. Soluble mesothelin-related peptide level elevation in mesothelioma serum and pleural effusions. Ann Thorac Surg 2008;85:265–72 [discussion: 272].

44. Amati M, Tomasetti M, Scartozzi M, et al. Profiling tumor-associated markers for early detection of malignant mesothelioma: an epidemiologic study. Cancer Epidemiol Biomarkers Prev 2008;17:163–70.

45. Scherpereel A, Grigoriu B, Conti M, et al. Soluble mesothelin-related peptides in the diagnosis of malignant pleural mesothelioma. Am J Respir Crit Care Med 2006;173:1155–60.

46. Rodriguez Portal JA, Rodriguez Becerra E, Rodriguez Rodriguez D, et al. Serum levels of soluble mesothelin-related peptides in malignant and nonmalignant asbestos-related pleural disease: relation with past asbestos exposure. Cancer Epidemiol Biomarkers Prev 2009;18:646–50.

47. Hassan R, Remaley AT, Sampson ML, et al. Detection and quantitation of serum mesothelin, a tumor marker for patients with mesothelioma and ovarian cancer. Clin Cancer Res 2006;12:447–53.

48. Luo L, Shi HZ, Liang QL, et al. Diagnostic value of soluble mesothelin-related peptides for malignant mesothelioma: a meta-analysis. Respir Med 2010;104:149–56.

49. Hollevoet K, Reitsma JB, Creaney J, et al. Serum mesothelin for diagnosing malignant pleural mesothelioma: an individual patient data meta-analysis. J Clin Oncol 2012;30:1541–9.

50. Filiberti R, Marroni P, Mencoboni M, et al. Individual predictors of increased serum mesothelin in asbestos-exposed workers. Med Oncol 2013;30:422.

51. Park EK, Sandrini A, Yates DH, et al. Soluble mesothelin-related protein in an asbestos-exposed population: the Dust Diseases Board cohort study. Am J Respir Crit Care Med 2008;178:832–7.

52. Hollevoet K, Nackaerts K, Gosselin R, et al. Soluble mesothelin, megakaryocyte potentiating factor, and osteopontin as markers of patient response and outcome in mesothelioma. J Thorac Oncol 2011;6:1930–7.

53. Pass HI, Brewer GJ, Dick R, et al. A phase II trial of tetrathiomolybdate after surgery for malignant

mesothelioma: final results. Ann Thorac Surg 2008; 86:383–9 [discussion: 390].

54. Burt BM, Lee HS, Lenge De Rosen V, et al. Soluble mesothelin-related peptides to monitor recurrence after resection of pleural mesothelioma. Ann Thorac Surg 2017;104:1679–87.

55. Hollevoet K, Van Cleemput J, Thimpont J, et al. Serial measurements of mesothelioma serum biomarkers in asbestos-exposed individuals: a prospective longitudinal cohort study. J Thorac Oncol 2011;6:889–95.

56. Wheatley-Price P, Yang B, Patsios D, et al. Soluble mesothelin-related peptide and osteopontin as markers of response in malignant mesothelioma. J Clin Oncol 2010;28:3316–22.

57. Creaney J, Francis RJ, Dick IM, et al. Serum soluble mesothelin concentrations in malignant pleural mesothelioma: relationship to tumor volume, clinical stage and changes in tumor burden. Clin Cancer Res 2011;17:1181–9.

58. Linch M, Gennatas S, Kazikin S, et al. A serum mesothelin level is a prognostic indicator for patients with malignant mesothelioma in routine clinical practice. BMC Cancer 2014;14:674.

59. Schneider J, Hoffmann H, Dienemann H, et al. Diagnostic and prognostic value of soluble mesothelin-related proteins in patients with malignant pleural mesothelioma in comparison with benign asbestosis and lung cancer. J Thorac Oncol 2008;3:1317–24.

60. Cristaudo A, Foddis R, Vivaldi A, et al. Clinical significance of serum mesothelin in patients with mesothelioma and lung cancer. Clin Cancer Res 2007;13:5076–81.

61. Grigoriu BD, Scherpereel A, Devos P, et al. Utility of osteopontin and serum mesothelin in malignant pleural mesothelioma diagnosis and prognosis assessment. Clin Cancer Res 2007;13:2928–35.

62. Tian L, Zeng R, Wang X, et al. Prognostic significance of soluble mesothelin in malignant pleural mesothelioma: a meta-analysis. Oncotarget 2017; 8:46425–35.

63. Hollevoet K, Nackaerts K, Thas O, et al. The effect of clinical covariates on the diagnostic and prognostic value of soluble mesothelin and megakaryocyte potentiating factor. Chest 2012;141:477–84.

64. Creaney J, Dick IM, Meniawy TM, et al. Comparison of fibulin-3 and mesothelin as markers in malignant mesothelioma. Thorax 2014;69:895–902.

65. de Fonseka D, Arnold DT, Stadon L, et al. A prospective study to investigate the role of serial serum mesothelin in monitoring mesothelioma. BMC cancer 2018;18:199.

66. Arnold DT, De Fonseka D, Hamilton FW, et al. Prognostication and monitoring of mesothelioma using biomarkers: a systematic review. Br J Cancer 2017;116:731–41.

67. Shiomi K, Miyamoto H, Segawa T, et al. Novel ELISA system for detection of N-ERC/mesothelin in the sera of mesothelioma patients. Cancer Sci 2006;97:928–32.

68. Onda M, Nagata S, Ho M, et al. Megakaryocyte potentiation factor cleaved from mesothelin precursor is a useful tumor marker in the serum of patients with mesothelioma. Clin Cancer Res 2006;12: 4225–31.

69. Hollevoet K, Nackaerts K, Thimpont J, et al. Diagnostic performance of soluble mesothelin and megakaryocyte potentiating factor in mesothelioma. Am J Respir Crit Care Med 2010;181:620–5.

70. Park EK, Thomas PS, Creaney J, et al. Factors affecting soluble mesothelin related protein levels in an asbestos-exposed population. Clin Chem Lab Med 2010;48:869–74.

71. Shiomi K, Shiomi S, Ishinaga Y, et al. Impact of renal failure on the tumor markers of mesothelioma, N-ERC/mesothelin and osteopontin. Anticancer Res 2011;31:1427–30.

72. Wai PY, Kuo PC. The role of osteopontin in tumor metastasis. J Surg Res 2004;121:228–41.

73. Chen RX, Xia YH, Xue TC, et al. Osteopontin promotes hepatocellular carcinoma invasion by up-regulating MMP-2 and uPA expression. Mol Biol Rep 2011;38:3671–7.

74. Tajima K, Ohashi R, Sekido Y, et al. Osteopontin-mediated enhanced hyaluronan binding induces multidrug resistance in mesothelioma cells. Oncogene 2010;29:1941–51.

75. Ohashi R, Tajima K, Takahashi F, et al. Osteopontin modulates malignant pleural mesothelioma cell functions in vitro. Anticancer Res 2009;29: 2205–14.

76. Frey AB, Wali A, Pass H, et al. Osteopontin is linked to p65 and MMP-9 expression in pulmonary adenocarcinoma but not in malignant pleural mesothelioma. Histopathology 2007;50:720–6.

77. Coppola D, Szabo M, Boulware D, et al. Correlation of osteopontin protein expression and pathological stage across a wide variety of tumor histologies. Clin Cancer Res 2004;10:184–90.

78. Rouanne M, Adam J, Goubar A, et al. Osteopontin and thrombospondin-1 play opposite roles in promoting tumor aggressiveness of primary resected non-small cell lung cancer. BMC Cancer 2016;16:483.

79. El-Tanani MK, Yuen HF, Shi Z, et al. Osteopontin can act as an effector for a germline mutation of BRCA1 in malignant transformation of breast cancer-related cells. Cancer Sci 2010;101: 1354–60.

80. Pass HI, Lott D, Lonardo F, et al. Asbestos exposure, pleural mesothelioma, and serum osteopontin levels. N Engl J Med 2005;353:1564–73.

81. Ivanov SV, Ivanova AV, Goparaju CM, et al. Tumorigenic properties of alternative osteopontin

isoforms in mesothelioma. Biochem Biophys Res Commun 2009;382:514–8.

82. Felten MK, Khatab K, Knoll L, et al. Changes of mesothelin and osteopontin levels over time in formerly asbestos-exposed power industry workers. Int Arch Occup Environ Health 2014;87: 195–204.

83. Sandhu H, Dehnen W, Roller M, et al. mRNA expression patterns in different stages of asbestos-induced carcinogenesis in rats. Carcinogenesis 2000;21:1023–9.

84. Cristaudo A, Bonotti A, Simonini S, et al. Combined serum mesothelin and plasma osteopontin measurements in malignant pleural mesothelioma. J Thorac Oncol 2011;6:1587–93.

85. Cristaudo A, Foddis R, Bonotti A, et al. Comparison between plasma and serum osteopontin levels: usefulness in diagnosis of epithelial malignant pleural mesothelioma. Int J Biol Markers 2010;25: 164–70.

86. Rai AJ, Flores RM, Mathew A, et al. Soluble mesothelin related peptides (SMRP) and osteopontin as protein biomarkers for malignant mesothelioma: analytical validation of ELISA based assays and characterization at mRNA and protein levels. Clin Chem Lab Med 2010;48:271–8.

87. Paleari L, Rotolo N, Imperatori A, et al. Osteopontin is not a specific marker in malignant pleural mesothelioma. Int J Biol Markers 2009;24:112–7.

88. Creaney J, Yeoman D, Musk AW, et al. Plasma versus serum levels of osteopontin and mesothelin in patients with malignant mesothelioma—which is best? Lung Cancer 2011;74:55–60.

89. Hu ZD, Liu XF, Liu XC, et al. Diagnostic accuracy of osteopontin for malignant pleural mesothelioma: a systematic review and meta-analysis. Clin Chim Acta 2014;433:44–8.

90. Cappia S, Righi L, Mirabelli D, et al. Prognostic role of osteopontin expression in malignant pleural mesothelioma. Am J Clin Pathol 2008; 130:58–64.

91. Pass HI, Goparaju C, Espin-Garcia O, et al. Plasma biomarker enrichment of clinical prognostic indices in malignant pleural mesothelioma. J Thorac Oncol 2016;11:900–9.

92. Bruno F, Baratti D, Martinetti A, et al. Mesothelin and osteopontin as circulating markers of diffuse malignant peritoneal mesothelioma: A preliminary study. Eur J Surg Oncol 2018;44:792–8.

93. Bonotti A, Simonini S, Pantani E, et al. Serum mesothelin, osteopontin and vimentin: useful markers for clinical monitoring of malignant pleural mesothelioma. Int J Biol Markers 2017;32:e126–31.

94. Obaya AJ, Rua S, Moncada-Pazos A, et al. The dual role of fibulins in tumorigenesis. Cancer Lett 2012;325:132–8.

95. Zhang Y, Marmorstein LY. Focus on molecules: fibulin-3 (EFEMP1). Exp Eye Res 2010;90:374–5.

96. Pass HI, Levin SM, Harbut MR, et al. Fibulin-3 as a blood and effusion biomarker for pleural mesothelioma. N Engl J Med 2012;367:1417–27.

97. Agha MA, El-Habashy MM, El-Shazly RA. Role of fibulin-3 in the diagnosis of malignant mesothelioma. Egypt J Chest Dis Tuberc 2014;63:99–105.

98. Demir M, Kaya H, Taylan M, et al. Evaluation of new biomarkers in the prediction of malignant mesothelioma in subjects with environmental asbestos exposure. Lung 2016;194:409–17.

99. Jiang Z, Ying S, Shen W, et al. Plasma fibulin-3 as a potential biomarker for patients with asbestos-related diseases in the han population. Dis markers 2017;2017:1725354.

100. Kaya H, Demir M, Taylan M, et al. Fibulin-3 as a diagnostic biomarker in patients with malignant mesothelioma. Asian Pac J Cancer Prev 2015;16: 1403–7.

101. Kirschner MB, Pulford E, Hoda MA, et al. Fibulin-3 levels in malignant pleural mesothelioma are associated with prognosis but not diagnosis. Br J Cancer 2015;113:963–9.

102. Battolla E, Canessa PA, Ferro P, et al. Comparison of the diagnostic performance of fibulin-3 and mesothelin in patients with pleural effusions from malignant mesothelioma. Anticancer Res 2017;37: 1387–91.

103. Pei D, Li Y, Liu X, et al. Diagnostic and prognostic utilities of humoral fibulin-3 in malignant pleural mesothelioma: evidence from a meta-analysis. Oncotarget 2017;8:13030–8.

104. Nandhu MS, Behera P, Bhaskaran V, et al. Development of a function-blocking antibody against fibulin-3 as a targeted reagent for glioblastoma. Clin Cancer Res 2018;24:821–33.

105. Borrebaeck CA. Precision diagnostics: moving towards protein biomarker signatures of clinical utility in cancer. Nat Rev Cancer 2017;17: 199–204.

106. Giusti L, Da Valle Y, Bonotti A, et al. Comparative proteomic analysis of malignant pleural mesothelioma evidences an altered expression of nuclear lamin and filament-related proteins. Proteomics Clin Appl 2014;8:258–68.

107. Ostroff RM, Mehan MR, Stewart A, et al. Early detection of malignant pleural mesothelioma in asbestos-exposed individuals with a noninvasive proteomics-based surveillance tool. PLoS One 2012;7:e46091.

108. Kraemer S, Vaught JD, Bock C, et al. From SOMAmer-based biomarker discovery to diagnostic and clinical applications: a SOMAmer-based, streamlined multiplex proteomic assay. PLoS One 2011;6:e26332.

109. Gold L, Ayers D, Bertino J, et al. Aptamer-based multiplexed proteomic technology for biomarker discovery. PLoS One 2010;5:e15004.

110. White R, Pulford E, Elliot DJ, et al. Quantitative mass spectrometry to identify protein markers for diagnosis of malignant pleural mesothelioma. J Proteomics 2019;192:374–82.

111. Cerciello F, Choi M, Nicastri A, et al. Identification of a seven glycopeptide signature for malignant pleural mesothelioma in human serum by selected reaction monitoring. Clin Proteomics 2013;10:16.

112. Greening DW, Ji H, Chen M, et al. Secreted primary human malignant mesothelioma exosome signature reflects oncogenic cargo. Sci Rep 2016;6: 32643.

113. Pass HI, Liu Z, Wali A, et al. Gene expression profiles predict survival and progression of pleural mesothelioma. Clin Cancer Res 2004;10(3):849–59.

114. Gordon GJ, Dong L, Yeap BY, et al. Four-gene expression ratio test for survival in patients undergoing surgery for mesothelioma. J Natl Cancer Inst 2009;101:678–86.

115. Gordon GJ, Jensen RV, Hsiao LL, et al. Using gene expression ratios to predict outcome among patients with mesothelioma. J Natl Cancer Inst 2003; 95:598–605.

116. Gordon GJ, Rockwell GN, Godfrey PA, et al. Validation of genomics-based prognostic tests in malignant pleural mesothelioma. Clin Cancer Res 2005;11:4406–14.

117. Gill RR, Yeap BY, Bueno R, et al. Quantitative Clinical staging for patients with malignant pleural mesothelioma. J Natl Cancer Inst 2018;110: 258–64.

118. Zhou J-G, Zhong H, Zhang J, et al. Development and validation of a prognostic signature for malignant pleural mesothelioma. Front Oncol 2019;9: 78.

119. Ivanov SV, Miller J, Lucito R, et al. Genomic events associated with progression of pleural malignant mesothelioma. Int J Cancer 2009;124:589–99.

120. Bueno R, Stawiski EW, Goldstein LD, et al. Comprehensive genomic analysis of malignant pleural mesothelioma identifies recurrent mutations, gene fusions and splicing alterations. Nat Genet 2016;48:407–16.

121. Hmeljak J, Sanchez-Vega F, Hoadley KA, et al. Integrative molecular characterization of malignant pleural mesothelioma. Cancer Discov 2018;8: 1548–65.

122. Testa JR, Cheung M, Pei J, et al. Germline BAP1 mutations predispose to malignant mesothelioma. Nat Genet 2011;43:1022–5.

123. Carbone M, Yang H, Pass HI, et al. BAP1 and cancer. Nat Rev Cancer 2013;13:153–9.

124. Pastorino S, Yoshikawa Y, Pass HI, et al. A subset of mesotheliomas with improved survival occurring in carriers of BAP1 and other germline mutations. J Clin Oncol 2018;36(35). JCO2018790352.

125. Arzt L, Quehenberger F, Halbwedl I, et al. BAP1 protein is a progression factor in malignant pleural mesothelioma. Pathol Oncol Res 2014;20:145–51.

126. López-Ríos F, Chuai S, Flores R, et al. Global gene expression profiling of pleural mesotheliomas: overexpression of aurora kinases and P16/ CDKN2A deletion as prognostic factors and critical evaluation of microarray-based prognostic prediction. Cancer Res 2006;66:2970–9.

127. Dacic S, Kothmaier H, Land S, et al. Prognostic significance of p16/cdkn2a loss in pleural malignant mesotheliomas. Virchows Arch 2008;453:627–35.

128. Chou A, Toon CW, Clarkson A, et al. The epithelioid BAP1-negative and p16-positive phenotype predicts prolonged survival in pleural mesothelioma. Histopathology 2018;72:509–15.

129. Di Leva G, Garofalo M, Croce CM. MicroRNAs in cancer. Annu Rev Pathol 2014;9:287–314.

130. Ambros V. The functions of animal microRNAs. Nature 2004;431:350–5.

131. Bartel DP. MicroRNAs: genomics, biogenesis, mechanism, and function. Cell 2004;116:281–97.

132. Griffiths-Jones S. miRBase: the microRNA sequence database. Methods Mol Biol 2006;342: 129–38.

133. Reddy KB. MicroRNA (miRNA) in cancer. Cancer Cell Int 2015;15:38.

134. Reid G. MicroRNAs in mesothelioma: from tumour suppressors and biomarkers to therapeutic targets. J Thorac Dis 2015;7:1031–40.

135. Li MH, Fu SB, Xiao HS. Genome-wide analysis of microRNA and mRNA expression signatures in cancer. Acta Pharmacol Sin 2015;36:1200–11.

136. Lamberti M, Capasso R, Lombardi A, et al. Two different serum MiRNA signatures correlate with the clinical outcome and histological subtype in pleural malignant mesothelioma patients. PLoS One 2015;10:e0135331.

137. Weber DG, Casjens S, Johnen G, et al. Combination of MiR-103a-3p and mesothelin improves the biomarker performance of malignant mesothelioma diagnosis. PLoS One 2014;9:e114483.

138. Kirschner MB, Cheng YY, Badrian B, et al. Increased circulating miR-625-3p: a potential biomarker for patients with malignant pleural mesothelioma. J Thorac Oncol 2012;7:1184–91.

139. Busacca S, Germano S, De Cecco L, et al. MicroRNA signature of malignant mesothelioma with potential diagnostic and prognostic implications. Am J Respir Cell Mol Biol 2010;42:312–9.

140. Guled M, Lahti L, Lindholm PM, et al. CDKN2A, NF2, and JUN are dysregulated among other genes by miRNAs in malignant mesothelioma—a miRNA microarray analysis. Genes Chromosomes Cancer 2009;48:615–23.

141. Pass HI, Goparaju C, Ivanov S, et al. hsa-miR-29c* is linked to the prognosis of malignant pleural mesothelioma. Cancer Res 2010;70:1916–24.

142. Ivanov SV, Goparaju CM, Lopez P, et al. Pro-tumorigenic effects of miR-31 loss in mesothelioma. J Biol Chem 2010;285:22809–17.

143. Tomasetti M, Staffolani S, Nocchi L, et al. Clinical significance of circulating miR-126 quantification in malignant mesothelioma patients. Clin Biochem 2012;45:575–81.

144. Santarelli L, Staffolani S, Strafella E, et al. Combined circulating epigenetic markers to improve mesothelin performance in the diagnosis of malignant mesothelioma. Lung Cancer 2015;90:457–64.

145. Micolucci L, Akhtar MM, Olivieri F, et al. Diagnostic value of microRNAs in asbestos exposure and malignant mesothelioma: systematic review and qualitative meta-analysis. Oncotarget 2016;7: 58606–37.

146. Lo Russo G, Tessari A, Capece M, et al. MicroRNAs for the diagnosis and management of malignant pleural mesothelioma: a literature review. Front Oncol 2018;8:650.

147. Mozzoni P, Ampollini L, Goldoni M, et al. MicroRNA expression in malignant pleural mesothelioma and asbestosis: a pilot study. Dis Markers 2017;2017: 9645940.

148. Andersen M, Grauslund M, Ravn J, et al. Diagnostic potential of miR-126, miR-143, miR-145, and miR-652 in malignant pleural mesothelioma. J Mol Diagn 2014;16:418–30.

149. Matboli M, Shafei AE, Azazy AE, et al. Clinical evaluation of circulating miR-548a-3p and -20a expression in malignant pleural mesothelioma patients. Biomark Med 2018;12:129–39.

150. Sun JG, Pass H. MicroRNAs for Diagnosis and Prognosis of Mesothelioma. In Poster Presentation Edition. San Diego, CA: AATS Annual Meeting, April 28 - May 1, 2018.

151. Bononi I, Comar M, Puozzo A, et al. Circulating microRNAs found dysregulated in ex-exposed asbestos workers and pleural mesothelioma patients as potential new biomarkers. Oncotarget 2016;7:82700–11.

152. Cavalleri T, Angelici L, Favero C, et al. Plasmatic extracellular vesicle microRNAs in malignant pleural mesothelioma and asbestos-exposed subjects suggest a 2-miRNA signature as potential biomarker of disease. PLoS One 2017;12: e0176680.

153. Weber DG, Johnen G, Bryk O, et al. Identification of miRNA-103 in the cellular fraction of human peripheral blood as a potential biomarker for malignant mesothelioma—a pilot study. PLoS One 2012;7:e30221.

154. Matboli M, Shafei AE, Ali MA, et al. Clinical significance of serum DRAM1 mRNA, ARSA mRNA, hsa-miR-2053 and lncRNA-RP1-86D1.3 axis expression in malignant pleural mesothelioma. J Cell Biochem 2019;120:3203–11.

155. Matsumoto S, Nabeshima K, Hamasaki M, et al. Upregulation of microRNA-31 associates with a poor prognosis of malignant pleural mesothelioma with sarcomatoid component. Med Oncol 2014; 31:303.

156. Fassina A, Cappellesso R, Guzzardo V, et al. Epithelial-mesenchymal transition in malignant mesothelioma. Mod Pathol 2012;25:86–99.

157. Kirschner MB, Cheng YY, Armstrong NJ, et al. MiR-score: a novel 6-microRNA signature that predicts survival outcomes in patients with malignant pleural mesothelioma. Mol Oncol 2015;9: 715–26.

158. De Santi C, Melaiu O, Bonotti A, et al. Deregulation of miRNAs in malignant pleural mesothelioma is associated with prognosis and suggests an alteration of cell metabolism. Sci Rep 2017;7:3140.

159. Andersen M, Trapani D, Ravn J, et al. Methylation-associated silencing of microRNA-126 and its host gene EGFL7 in malignant pleural mesothelioma. Anticancer Res 2015;35:6223–9.

160. Johnson TG, Schelch K, Cheng YY, et al. Dysregulated expression of the microRNA miR-137 and its target YBX1 contribute to the invasive characteristics of malignant pleural mesothelioma. J Thorac Oncol 2018;13:258–72.

161. Mairinger FD, Werner R, Flom E, et al. miRNA regulation is important for DNA damage repair and recognition in malignant pleural mesothelioma. Virchows Arch 2017;470:627–37.

162. De Rubis G, Rajeev Krishnan S, Bebawy M. Liquid biopsies in cancer diagnosis, monitoring, and prognosis. Trends Pharmacol Sci 2019;40:172–86.

163. Corcoran RB, Chabner BA. Application of cell-free DNA analysis to cancer treatment. N Engl J Med 2018;379:1754–65.

164. Leon SA, Shapiro B, Sklaroff DM, et al. Free DNA in the serum of cancer patients and the effect of therapy. Cancer Res 1977;37:646–50.

165. Hylebos M, Op de Beeck K, Pauwels P, et al. Tumor-specific genetic variants can be detected in circulating cell-free DNA of malignant pleural mesothelioma patients. Lung Cancer 2018;124:19–22.

166. Muraoka T, Soh J, Toyooka S, et al. The degree of microRNA-34b/c methylation in serum-circulating DNA is associated with malignant pleural mesothelioma. Lung Cancer 2013;82:485–90.

167. Sato H, Soh J, Aoe K, et al. Droplet digital PCR as a novel system for the detection of microRNA34b/c methylation in circulating DNA in malignant pleural mesothelioma. Int J Oncol 2019;54:2139–48.

168. Moore LD, Le T, Fan G. DNA methylation and its basic function. Neuropsychopharmacology 2013; 38:23–38.

169. Vandermeers F, Neelature Sriramareddy S, Costa C, et al. The role of epigenetics in malignant pleural mesothelioma. Lung Cancer 2013;81: 311–8.

170. Guarrera S, Viberti C, Cugliari G, et al. Peripheral blood DNA methylation as potential biomarker of malignant pleural mesothelioma in asbestos-exposed subjects. J Thorac Oncol 2019;14: 527–39.

171. Huang H, Shi Y, Huang J, et al. Circulating tumor cells as a potential biomarker in diagnosis of lung cancer: a systematic review and meta-analysis. Clin Respir J 2018;12:639–45.

172. Raphael J, Massard C, Gong IY, et al. Detection of circulating tumour cells in peripheral blood of patients with malignant pleural mesothelioma. Cancer Biomark 2015;15:151–6.

173. Yoneda K, Tanaka F, Kondo N, et al. Circulating tumor cells (CTCs) in malignant pleural mesothelioma (MPM). Ann Surg Oncol 2014;21(Suppl 4): S472–80.

174. Chikaishi Y, Yoneda K, Ohnaga T, et al. EpCAM-independent capture of circulating tumor cells with a 'universal CTC-chip. Oncol Rep 2017;37:77–82.

175. Scaffidi P, Misteli T, Bianchi ME. Release of chromatin protein HMGB1 by necrotic cells triggers inflammation. Nature 2002;418:191–5.

176. Bianchi ME, Beltrame M, Paonessa G. Specific recognition of cruciform DNA by nuclear protein HMG1. Science 1989;243:1056–9.

177. Venereau E, Ceriotti C, Bianchi ME. DAMPs from cell death to new life. Front Immunol 2015;6:422.

178. Lu B, Antoine DJ, Kwan K, et al. JAK/STAT1 signaling promotes HMGB1 hyperacetylation and nuclear translocation. Proc Natl Acad Sci U S A 2014;111:3068–73.

179. Carneiro VC, de Moraes Maciel R, de Abreu da Silva IC, et al. The extracellular release of *Schistosoma mansoni* HMGB1 nuclear protein is mediated by acetylation. Biochem Biophys Res Commun 2009;390:1245–9.

180. Jube S, Rivera ZS, Bianchi ME, et al. Cancer cell secretion of the DAMP protein HMGB1 supports progression in malignant mesothelioma. Cancer Res 2012;72:3290–301.

181. Wang Y, Faux SP, Hallden G, et al. Interleukin-1beta and tumour necrosis factor-alpha promote the transformation of human immortalised mesothelial cells by erionite. Int J Oncol 2004;25:173–8.

182. Ying S, Jiang Z, He X, et al. Serum HMGB1 as a potential biomarker for patients with asbestos-related diseases. Dis Markers 2017;2017:5756102.

183. Napolitano A, Antoine DJ, Pellegrini L, et al. HMGB1 and its hyperacetylated isoform are sensitive and specific serum biomarkers to detect asbestos exposure and to identify mesothelioma patients. Clin Cancer Res 2016;22:3087–96.

184. Wu T, Zhang W, Yang G, et al. HMGB1 overexpression as a prognostic factor for survival in cancer: a meta-analysis and systematic review. Oncotarget 2016;7:50417–27.

185. Yamagishi T, Fujimoto N, Nishi H, et al. Prognostic significance of the lymphocyte-to-monocyte ratio in patients with malignant pleural mesothelioma. Lung Cancer 2015;90:111–7.

186. Kao SCH, Pavlakis N, Harvie R, et al. High blood neutrophil-to-lymphocyte ratio is an indicator of poor prognosis in malignant mesothelioma patients undergoing systemic therapy. Clin Cancer Res 2010;16:5805–13.

187. Kao SC-H, Klebe S, Henderson DW, et al. Low calretinin expression and high neutrophil-to-lymphocyte ratio are poor prognostic factors in patients with malignant mesothelioma undergoing extrapleural pneumonectomy. J Thorac Oncol 2011;6: 1923–9.

188. Pinato DJ, Mauri FA, Ramakrishnan R, et al. Inflammation-based prognostic indices in malignant pleural mesothelioma. J Thorac Oncol 2012;7: 587–94.

189. Kao SC, Vardy J, Chatfield M, et al. Validation of prognostic factors in malignant pleural mesothelioma: a retrospective analysis of data from patients seeking compensation from the New South Wales Dust Diseases Board. Clin Lung Cancer 2013;14: 70–7.

190. Meniawy TM, Creaney J, Lake RA, et al. Existing models, but not neutrophil-to-lymphocyte ratio, are prognostic in malignant mesothelioma. Br J Cancer 2013;109:1813–20.

191. Cedrés S, Montero MA, Zamora E, et al. Expression of Wilms' tumor gene (WT1) is associated with survival in malignant pleural mesothelioma. Clin Transl Oncol 2014;16:776–82.

192. Klikovits T, Stockhammer P, Laszlo V, et al. Circulating complement component 4d (C4d) correlates with tumor volume, chemotherapeutic response and survival in patients with malignant pleural mesothelioma. Sci Rep 2017;7:16456.

193. Rogers JH. Calretinin: a gene for a novel calcium-binding protein expressed principally in neurons. J Cell Biol 1987;105:1343–53.

194. Schwaller B, Celio MR, Doglioni C. Identification of calretinin and the alternatively spliced form calretinin-22k in primary pleural mesotheliomas and in their metastases. Anticancer Res 2004;24: 4003–9.

195. Raiko I, Sander I, Weber DG, et al. Development of an enzyme-linked immunosorbent assay for the detection of human calretinin in plasma and serum of mesothelioma patients. BMC Cancer 2010;10:242.

196. Johnen G, Gawrych K, Raiko I, et al. Calretinin as a blood-based biomarker for mesothelioma. BMC Cancer 2017;17:386.

197. Aguilar-Madrid G, Pesch B, Calderon-Aranda ES, et al. Biomarkers for predicting malignant pleural mesothelioma in a Mexican population. Int J Med Sci 2018;15:883–91.

198. Casjens S, Weber DG, Johnen G, et al. Assessment of potential predictors of calretinin and mesothelin to improve the diagnostic performance to detect malignant mesothelioma: results from a population-based cohort study. BMJ Open 2017; 7:e017104.

199. Johnen G, Burek K, Raiko I, et al. Prediagnostic detection of mesothelioma by circulating calretinin and mesothelin—a case-control comparison nested into a prospective cohort of asbestos-exposed workers. Sci Rep 2018;8:14321.

200. Thapa B, Walkiewicz M, Murone C, et al. Calretinin but not caveolin-1 correlates with tumour histology and survival in malignant mesothelioma. Pathology 2016;48:660–5.

201. Morre DJ, Morre DM. Cell surface NADH oxidases (ECTO-NOX proteins) with roles in cancer, cellular time-keeping, growth, aging and neurodegenerative diseases. Free Radic Res 2003;37: 795–808.

202. Hostetler B, Weston N, Kim C, et al. Cancer site-specific isoforms of ENOX2 (tNOX), a cancer-specific cell surface oxidase. Clin Proteomics 2009;5:46–51.

203. Morré DJ, Hostetler B, Taggart DJ, et al. ENOX2-based early detection (ONCOblot) of asbestos-induced malignant mesothelioma 4–10 years in advance of clinical symptoms. Clin Proteomics 2016;13:2.

204. Cunningham GM, Roman MG, Flores LC, et al. The paradoxical role of thioredoxin on oxidative stress and aging. Arch Biochem Biophys 2015; 576:32–8.

205. Kumar-Singh S, Weyler J, Martin MJ, et al. Angiogenic cytokines in mesothelioma: a study of VEGF, FGF-1 and -2, and TGF beta expression. J Pathol 1999;189:72–8.

206. Strizzi L, Catalano A, Vianale G, et al. Vascular endothelial growth factor is an autocrine growth factor in human malignant mesothelioma. J Pathol 2001;193:468–75.

207. Demirag F, Unsal E, Yilmaz A, et al. Prognostic significance of vascular endothelial growth factor, tumor necrosis, and mitotic activity index in malignant pleural mesothelioma. Chest 2005;128: 3382–7.

208. Hirayama N, Tabata C, Tabata R, et al. Pleural effusion VEGF levels as a prognostic factor of malignant pleural mesothelioma. Respir Med 2011;105: 137–42.

209. Yasumitsu A, Tabata C, Tabata R, et al. Clinical significance of serum vascular endothelial growth factor in malignant pleural mesothelioma. J Thorac Oncol 2010;5:479–83.

210. Nowak AK, Millward MJ, Creaney J, et al. A phase II study of intermittent sunitinib malate as second-line therapy in progressive malignant pleural mesothelioma. J Thorac Oncol 2012;7:1449–56.

211. Stockhammer P, Ploenes T, Theegarten D, et al. Detection of TGF-β in pleural effusions for diagnosis and prognostic stratification of malignant pleural mesothelioma. Lung Cancer 2020;139: 124–32.

212. Vandooren J, Van den Steen PE, Opdenakker G. Biochemistry and molecular biology of gelatinase B or matrix metalloproteinase-9 (MMP-9): the next decade. Crit Rev Biochem Mol Biol 2013;48: 222–72.

213. Štrbac D, Goričar K, Dolžan V, et al. Matrix metalloproteinases polymorphisms as baseline risk predictors in malignant pleural mesothelioma. Radiol Oncol 2018;52:160–6.

214. Štrbac D, Goričar K, Dolžan V, et al. Matrix metalloproteinases polymorphisms as prognostic biomarkers in malignant pleural mesothelioma. Dis markers 2017;2017:8069529.

215. Štrbac D, Goričar K, Dolžan V, et al. Evaluation of matrix metalloproteinase 9 serum concentration as a biomarker in malignant mesothelioma. Dis markers 2019;2019:1242964.

216. Hong T-T, Smyth JW, Gao D, et al. BIN1 localizes the L-type calcium channel to cardiac T-tubules. PLoS Biol 2010;8:e1000312.

217. Ahmadzada T, Lee K, Clarke C, et al. High BIN1 expression has a favorable prognosis in malignant pleural mesothelioma and is associated with tumor infiltrating lymphocytes. Lung Cancer 2019;130: 35–41.

218. Peroza EA, Schmucki R, Güntert P, et al. The beta(E)-domain of wheat E(c)-1 metallothionein: a metal-binding domain with a distinctive structure. J Mol Biol 2009;387:207–18.

219. Mairinger FD, Schmeller J, Borchert S, et al. Immunohistochemically detectable metallothionein expression in malignant pleural mesotheliomas is strongly associated with early failure to platin-based chemotherapy. Oncotarget 2018;9: 22254–68.

220. Day RE, Kitchen P, Owen DS, et al. Human aquaporins: regulators of transcellular water flow. Biochim Biophys Acta 2014;1840:1492–506.

221. Angelico G, Caltabiano R, Loreto C, et al. Immunohistochemical expression of aquaporin-1 in fluoro-edenite-induced malignant mesothelioma: a preliminary report. Int J Mol Sci 2018;19:685.

222. Angelico G, Ieni A, Caltabiano R, et al. Aquaporin-1 expression in fluoro-edenite-induced mesothelioma effusions: an approach by cell-block procedure. Cytopathology 2018;29:455–60.

223. Marcq E, Waele JD, Audenaerde JV, et al. Abundant expression of TIM-3, LAG-3, PD-1 and PD-

L1 as immunotherapy checkpoint targets in effusions of mesothelioma patients. Oncotarget 2017; 8:89722–35.

224. Sobhani N, Roviello G, Pivetta T, et al. Tumour infiltrating lymphocytes and PD-L1 expression as potential predictors of outcome in patients with malignant pleural mesothelioma. Mol Biol Rep 2019;46:2713–20.

225. Nguyen BH, Montgomery R, Fadia M, et al. PD-L1 expression associated with worse survival outcome in malignant pleural mesothelioma. Asia Pac J Clin Oncol 2018;14:69–73.

226. Inaguma S, Lasota J, Wang Z, et al. Expression of ALCAM (CD166) and PD-L1 (CD274) independently predicts shorter survival in malignant pleural mesothelioma. Hum Pathol 2018;71:1–7.

227. Jimenez-Ramirez C, Casjens S, Juarez-Perez CA, et al. Mesothelin, calretinin, and megakaryocyte potentiating factor as biomarkers of malignant pleural mesothelioma. Lung 2019;197:641–9.

228. Bonotti A, Foddis R, Landi S, et al. A novel panel of serum biomarkers for MPM diagnosis. Dis Markers 2017;2017:3510984.

229. Doi H, Kuribayashi K, Kitajima K, et al. Development of a novel prognostic risk classification system for malignant pleural mesothelioma. Clin Lung Cancer 2020;21:66–74.e62.

230. Boots AW, van Berkel JJ, Dallinga JW, et al. The versatile use of exhaled volatile organic compounds in human health and disease. J Breath Res 2012;6:027108.

231. Ahmed WM, Lawal O, Nijsen TM, et al. Exhaled volatile organic compounds of infection: a systematic review. ACS Infect Dis 2017;3:695–710.

232. Lamote K, Nackaerts K, van Meerbeeck JP. Strengths, weaknesses, and opportunities of diagnostic breathomics in pleural mesothelioma—a hypothesis. Cancer Epidemiol Biomarkers Prev 2014; 23:898–908.

233. van Oort PM, Povoa P, Schnabel R, et al. The potential role of exhaled breath analysis in the diagnostic process of pneumonia—a systematic review. J Breath Res 2018;12:024001.

234. Brusselmans L, Arnouts L, Millevert C, et al. Breath analysis as a diagnostic and screening tool for malignant pleural mesothelioma: a systematic review. Transl Lung Cancer Res 2018;7:520–36.

235. Azim A, Barber C, Dennison P, et al. Exhaled volatile organic compounds in adult asthma: a systematic review. Eur Respir J 2019;54.

236. Amann A, Miekisch W, Schubert J, et al. Analysis of exhaled breath for disease detection. Annu Rev Anal Chem (Palo Alto Calif) 2014;7:455–82.

237. Smith D, Spanel P. Ambient analysis of trace compounds in gaseous media by SIFT-MS. Analyst 2011;136:2009–32.

238. Lamote K, Vynck M, Thas O, et al. Exhaled breath to screen for malignant pleural mesothelioma: a validation study. Eur Respir J 2017;50.

239. Bayram M, Dongel I, Akbas A, et al. Serum biomarkers in patients with mesothelioma and pleural plaques and healthy subjects exposed to naturally occurring asbestos. Lung 2014;192: 197–203.

The Staging of Malignant Pleural Mesothelioma

Caleb J. Euhus, MD, R. Taylor Ripley, MD*

KEYWORDS

- Staging • Malignant • Pleural mesothelioma • Lung cancer

KEY POINTS

- Malignant pleural mesothelioma (MPM) is an extensive tumor that spreads along the pleura and encases the lung. MPM spreads to pulmonary, mediastinal, and chest wall lymph nodes and occasionally to distant organs.
- Patients present at different times along this progression of disease, which is represented in the staging system for MPM.
- Based on the difficult of diagnosis and other tumors that mimic MPM, the staging system for MPM developed slowly until recently.

INTRODUCTION

Malignant pleural mesothelioma (MPM) is an extensive tumor that spreads along the pleura and encases the lung.[1] Initially, MPM forms small, independent nodules on the parietal pleura surface that convalesce into confluent sheets of tumor. The pleural space becomes obliterated and filled with effusions. As the tumor progresses, it invades chest wall, diaphragm, and pericardium as locally advanced disease. MPM spreads to pulmonary, mediastinal, and chest wall lymph nodes and occasionally to distant organs. Patients present at different times along this progression of disease, which is represented in the staging system for MPM.

Advances in staging of MPM have been hampered by the disease's rarity, late clinical presentation, and the nihilism secondary to poor outcomes regardless of treatment. Surgeons in the mid–twentieth century rarely encountered this disease. Patients who were evaluated usually presented in cardiopulmonary failure caused by complete encasement of all pleural surfaces. Despite Wagner and colleagues[2] establishing a link between asbestos exposure and a fatal cancer of the pleural in 1960, the histologic similarities between epithelial MPM and other diagnoses challenged pathologists and therefore delayed systematic staging.[3,4] Both primary and metastatic tumors of the pleural surface can mimic the pattern of spread of MPM. Lung adenocarcinoma can metastasizes along the pleura.[5] Extrathoracic primary tumors can metastasize to the pleura.[6] Epithelioid hemangioendothelioma is a rare tumor that closely mimics MPM.[7] Similarly, primary carcinoma and sarcoma originating from the pleura can occur. Based on the difficult of diagnosis and other tumors that mimic MPM, the staging system for MPM developed slowly until recently.

Before 1990, at least 5 staging systems were proposed for MPM: Butchart, Mattson, Sugarbaker, Chahinian, and the American Joint Committee on Cancer (AJCC).[8–13] These classification systems were mainly derived from single institutions, based on few cases, and were not externally validated. Whether tumor, node, and metastasis (TNM) descriptors were the basis for stages I through IV was variable. The systems were rarely applied, which hindered evaluation of whether they correlated well with patient survival.

In 1994, the International Association for the Study of Lung Cancer (IASLC) sponsored a workshop in London called the International

Department of Surgery, Division of General Thoracic Surgery, The Michael E. DeBakey Department of Surgery, Baylor College of Medicine, Houston, TX 77030, USA
* Corresponding author.
E-mail address: R.Taylor.Ripley@bcm.edu

Thorac Surg Clin 30 (2020) 425–433
https://doi.org/10.1016/j.thorsurg.2020.07.001
1547-4127/20/© 2020 Elsevier Inc. All rights reserved.

Mesothelioma Interest Group (IMIG).[8] This gathering of pulmonologists, thoracic surgeons, oncologists, epidemiologists, radiologists, pathologists, and laboratory scientists analyzed all of the available trials, reports, and databases covering MPM to create a universal staging system based on TNM descriptors. The proposed system was accepted by the Union for International Cancer Control (UICC) and AJCC as the international MPM staging system for the sixth and seventh editions of the staging manuals (**Table 1**). Shortly after it was adopted in 1996, the IMIG system was validated in 2 surgical series of MPM. Afterward, this system was applied to both retrospective series as well as prospective clinical trials.[14,15]

The system proposed by IMIG offered an international consensus for the staging of MPM but it still had several weaknesses. First, the system was derived from small studies with few patients. Second, most of series used in the system came from surgical reports; therefore, applying it to patients managed nonoperatively was difficult. Also, the type of operation performed for the disease influenced a patient's stage. Third, the system classified nodal disease based on lung cancer staging. Given that the nodal spread of MPM behaved differently than lung cancers, the usefulness of lung cancer staging for MPM was questionable even at the time of this proposal.

To further refine the IMIG 1994 staging system, IASLC and the Staging and Prognostic Factors Committee (SPFC) formed a database to collect anonymized MPM surgical cases. This effort was an international, multi-institutional cohort study that established a detailed database with broader representation of treatment modalities, new terminology, and an electronic data capture system. Cases with complete anatomic stage information, complete survival information, and diagnosis of MPM met eligibility criteria. Both clinical and pathologic staging information was obtained. Best stage was defined as pathologic stage when available after surgical resection; otherwise, clinical stage was considered as best stage. For patients who receive neoadjuvant chemotherapy, normally, the pathologic stage is denoted ypTNM, in which the y descriptor indicates the surgery was performed after chemotherapy. For the purposes of this study, only clinical staging was analyzed and ypTNM staging was not considered in these reports.

Surgeons from around the world leading programs with a high volume of patients with mesothelioma transferred data to the statistical center, Cancer Research and Biostatistics (CRAB), in Seattle, Washington. CRAB provided the biostatistical support for the analysis. Data for 3101 patients from 15 centers were collected from 1995 to 2009 and first published in 2012.[16] Data collection continued and ultimately 3519 cases from 29 centers on 4 continents were uploaded from January 1995 until June 2013. Cases after June 2013 were excluded to allow a minimum potential follow-up of 18 months by the time of analysis. The data were retrospectively added to the database for 1953 (55%) of the patients and prospectively collected for 1566 (45%) of the patients. Of the 3519 patients, 2460 passed the initial screening based on appropriate data elements and these patients were analyzed for the 2016 IASLC mesothelioma project. From this effort, formal revisions to the T, N, and M descriptors for the eighth edition of the TNM classification system were published. The most recent revisions are discussed later.

DISCUSSION
T Descriptors for Malignant Pleural Mesothelioma

The T descriptor in other solid tumors is often based on measurement of a concentrically growing primary lesion, which is prognostic of overall survival (OS). MPM's unusual rindlike growth pattern makes measurement for the T category difficult to generate. Therefore, the T category is based on spread from the pleura into other thoracic structures. In the eighth edition of the TNM classifications for pleural mesothelioma, T1 denotes disease limited to the ipsilateral pleura regardless of whether the involvement entails the parietal, visceral, diaphragmatic, or mediastinal pleura (**Table 2**). T2 signifies tumor of the pleural surfaces on the ipsilateral side in addition to involvement of the diaphragm muscle and/or extension into the pulmonary parenchyma. T3 involves invasion of all of the ipsilateral pleura but also has involvement of the endothoracic fascia, extension into the mediastinal fat, solitary resectable disease extending into the soft tissue of the chest wall, and/or nontransmural involvement of the pericardium. T4 involves all ipsilateral pleural surfaces with 1 or more of the following: diffuse extension or multifocal masses of tumor in the chest with or without rib destruction, direct transdiaphragmatic extension into the peritoneum, direct extension of tumor to the contralateral pleura, direct extension of tumor to mediastinal organs, tumor into the spine, and/or tumor extending through the internal surface of the pericardium with or without pericardial effusion with or without myocardial involvement. T3 disease is considered resectable, whereas T4 disease is considered unresectable. The IASLC mesothelioma project

Table 1
The 1995 international staging system for mesothelioma

Stage	Description
T1	T1a; tumor limited to the ipsilateral parietal pleura, including mediastinal and diaphragmatic pleura. No involvement of visceral pleura T1b: tumor involving the ipsilateral parietal pleura, including ipsilateral and diaphragmatic pleura. Scattered foci of tumor also involving the visceral pleura
T2	Tumor involving each of the ipsilateral pleural surfaces (parietal, mediastinal, diaphragmatic, and visceral) with at least 1 of the following features: • Involvement of diaphragmatic muscle • Confluent visceral pleural tumor (including the fissures) or extension of tumor from visceral pleura into the underlying pulmonary parenchyma
T3	Describes locally advanced but potentially resectable tumor. Tumor involving all of the ipsilateral pleural surfaces (parietal, mediastinal, diaphragmatic, and visceral) with at least 1 of the following features: • Involvement of the extrathoracic fascia • Extension into the mediastinal fat • Solitary, completely resectable focus of tumor extending into the soft tissues of the chest wall • Nontransmural involvement of the pericardium
T4	Describes locally advanced technically unresectable tumor. Tumor involving all of the ipsilateral pleural surfaces (parietal, mediastinal, diaphragmatic, and visceral) with at least 1 of the following features: • Diffuse extension or multifocal masses of tumor in the chest wall, with or without associated rib destruction • Direct transdiaphragmatic extension of tumor to the peritoneum • Direct extension of tumor to the contralateral pleura • Direct extension of tumor to 1 or more mediastinal organs • Direct extension of tumor into the spine • Tumor extending through to the internal surface of the pericardium with or without a pericardial effusion, or tumor involving the myocardium
N: Lymph Nodes	
NX	Regional lymph nodes cannot be assessed
N0	No lymph node metastases
N1	Metastases in the ipsilateral bronchopulmonary or hilar lymph nodes
N2	Metastases in the subcarinal or ipsilateral mediastinal lymph nodes, including the ipsilateral internal mammary nodes
N3	Metastases in the contralateral mediastinal, contralateral internal mammary, ipsilateral, or contralateral supraclavicular lymph node
M: Metastases	
mX	Presence of distant metastases cannot be assessed
m0	No distant metastases
M1	Distant metastases present
Stage	Description
Stage I	
1a	T1aN0M0
1b	T1bN0M0
Stage II	T2N0M0
Stage III	Any T3M0 Any N1M0 Any N2M0
Stage IV	Any T4 Any N3 Any M1

From Rusch VW. A proposed new international TNM staging system for malignant pleural mesothelioma from the International Mesothelioma Interest Group. Chest 1995;108(4):1125; with permission.

Table 2
The T descriptors for malignant pleural mesothelioma

T Component Staging	T Descriptors
TX	Primary tumor cannot be assessed
T0	No evidence of primary tumor
T1	Tumor limited to the ipsilateral parietal ± visceral ± mediastinal ± diaphragmatic pleura
T2	Tumor involving each of the ipsilateral pleural surfaces (parietal, mediastinal, diaphragmatic, and visceral pleura) with at least 1 of the following features: • Involvement of diaphragmatic muscle • Extension of tumor from visceral pleura into the underlying pulmonary parenchyma
T3	Describes locally advanced but potentially resectable tumor Tumor involving all of the ipsilateral pleural surfaces (parietal, mediastinal, diaphragmatic, and visceral pleura) with at least 1 of the following features: • Involvement of the endothoracic fascia • Extension into the mediastinal fat • Solitary, completely resectable focus of tumor extending into the soft tissues of the chest wall • Nontransmural involvement of the pericardium
T4	Describes locally advanced technically unresectable tumor Tumor involving all of the ipsilateral pleural surfaces (parietal, mediastinal, diaphragmatic, and visceral pleura) with at least 1 of the following features: • Diffuse extension or multifocal masses of tumor in the chest wall, with or without associated rib destruction • Direct transdiaphragmatic extension of tumor to the peritoneum • Direct extension of tumor to the contralateral pleura • Direct extension of tumor to mediastinal organs • Direct extension of tumor into the spine • Tumor extending through to the internal surface of the pericardium with or without a pericardial effusion; or tumor involving the myocardium

From Nowak AK, Chansky K, Rice DC, et al. The IASLC Mesothelioma Staging Project: proposals for revisions of the T descriptors in the forthcoming eighth edition of the TNM Classification for Pleural Mesothelioma. J Thorac Oncol. 2016;11(12):2095; with permission.

generated recommendations for the T descriptors based on clinical staging from 509 patients, pathologic staging from 836 patients, and both clinical and pathologic staging from 642 patients (**Fig. 1**).

In the analysis of clinical T staging, a separation in survival curves occurred between all categories except T1a and T1b.[17] However, no survival differences were noted from the pathologic staging between any of the T categories other than T3 and T4. Specifically, no difference in survival was noted between T1b, T2, or T3. In the previous staging system, T1 descriptor was divided into T1a and T1b based on involvement of ipsilateral parietal pleural without or with visceral pleural involvement, respectively. Given the poor discrimination between T1a and T1b on both clinical and pathologic staging, they were merged into a single T1 stage. Therefore, the distinction between

invasion of parietal and visceral pleura was eliminated. Given that nodal positivity is a strong predictor of survival, an adjustment for the N component was performed and did not change the results for outcomes based on the T component.

Comparison of clinical with pathologic T categories revealed that upstaging occurred frequently. Upstaging was recorded in 56% of clinical T1 patients, 54% of clinical T2 patients, and 39% of clinical T3 patients. Only 4% were assigned a lower pathologic stage than the clinical stage. Chest wall fascia, pericardium, or multiple T3 descriptors were the reasons that T1 or T2 were reclassified as T3. Multiple pathologic T4 descriptors were the reason for reclassifying T3 as T4. These findings suggest that clinical staging often underestimates the extent of the disease.

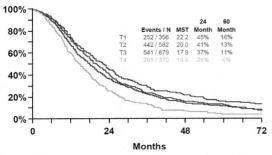

Fig. 1. OS of patients with malignant mesothelioma based on the best staging from the combination of clinical and pathologic T descriptors (see **Table 2**). (*From* Nowak AK, Chansky K, Rice DC, et al. The IASLC Mesothelioma Staging Project: proposals for revisions of the T descriptors in the forthcoming eighth edition of the TNM Classification for Pleural Mesothelioma. J Thorac Oncol. 2016;11(12):2094; with permission.)

Given the frequency that clinical T stage incorrectly predicted pathologic T stage as well as the unusually spread of MPM along pleural surfaces, tumor thickness was analyzed to ascertain its correlation with survival.[17] Measurements of pleural tumor thickness was available in 472 patients. Based on the sum of maximal thickness in upper, middle, and lower pleural measurements, quartiles were generated and survivals were compared as exploratory analyses. OS was inversely correlated with increasing thickness. A data-driven tumor cut point of 5.1 mm was identified. For a single maximal pleural thickness, median survivals of 24.2 and 17.7 months were noted when lesions were less than or greater than 5.1 mm, respectively. The patterns of tumor spread were also categorized as minimal, nodular, or rindlike, which revealed survivals of 23.4, 18.2, and 14.5 months,

respectively. Despite efforts to measure pleural thickness or categorize based on imaging patterns, these data are subject to a high degree of interobserver variability. Ultimately, computer-based volumetric analysis may systematize assessment of tumor mass into generating the T stage; however, this technology is not yet widespread enough to incorporate into the staging system. For the eighth edition of the staging system, tumor thickness is not a component of the T descriptor.

N Descriptors for Malignant Pleural Mesothelioma

In the eighth edition of the TNM classifications for pleural mesothelioma, N0 denotes absence of nodal metastasis (**Table 3**).[18] N1 signifies metastases to the ipsilateral bronchopulmonary, hilar, or mediastinal lymph nodes. The mediastinal lymph nodes include the internal mammary, peridiaphragmatic, pericardial fat pad, and the intercostal lymph nodes. N2 signifies the same nodal areas on the contralateral side in addition to both ipsilateral and contralateral supraclavicular lymph nodes. The IASLC mesothelioma project generated recommendations for the N descriptors based on clinical staging from 1603 patients, pathologic staging from 1614 patients, and both clinical and pathologic staging from 785 patients (**Fig. 2**).

In the prior staging system, nodal categories of N0 to N3 for MPM were adopted from the lung cancer staging.[8] Despite the recognition that the MPM lymphatic drainage is distinct from drainage in lung parenchymal tumors, this staging system remained for about 20 years. One problem with the lung cancer staging system arose from reports that questioned whether patients with pN1 and

Table 3
The N descriptors for malignant pleural mesothelioma

Regional Lymph Nodes(N)	Definition
NX	Regional lymph nodes cannot be assessed
N0	No regional lymph node metastases
N1	Metastases in the ipsilateral bronchopulmonary, hilar, or mediastinal (including the internal mammary, peridiaphragmatic, pericardial fat pad, or intercostal lymph nodes) lymph nodes
N2	Metastases in the contralateral bronchopulmonary, hilar, or mediastinal lymph nodes or ipsilateral or contralateral supraclavicular lymph nodes

From Rice D, Chansky K, Nowak A, et al. The IASLC Mesothelioma Staging Project: proposals for revisions of the N descriptors in the forthcoming eighth edition of the TNM Classification for Pleural Mesothelioma. J Thorac Oncol. 2016;11(12):2108; with permission.

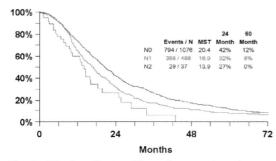

Fig. 2. OS of patients with malignant pleural mesothelioma based on the best staging from the combination of clinical and pathologic N descriptor (see **Table 3**). (*From* Rice D, Chansky K, Nowak A, et al. The IASLC Mesothelioma Staging Project: proposals for revisions of the N descriptors in the forthcoming eighth edition of the TNM Classification for Pleural Mesothelioma. J Thorac Oncol. 2016;11(12):2107; with permission. (Figure 7.C in original).)

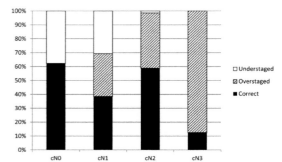

Fig. 3. The portion of patients whose N category was understaged, overstaged, or staged correctly when pathologic N staging is compared with clinical N staging. (*From* Rice D, Chansky K, Nowak A, et al. The IASLC Mesothelioma Staging Project: proposals for revisions of the N descriptors in the forthcoming eighth edition of the TNM Classification for Pleural Mesothelioma. J Thorac Oncol. 2016 Dec;11(12):2105; with permission.)

pN2 disease had different survivals.[16] Given that this limitation was known from the first adoption of the IMIG proposals, a data-driven IASLC database was the most anticipated component of this effort.

In total, 1328 patients had complete clinical staging and M0 disease.[18] Among these patients, 78% had cN0, 3% had cN1, 16% had cN2, and 3% had cN3. The median survivals for cN0, cN1, cN2, and cN3 were 19.0, 17.6, 16.2, and 14.5 months, respectively. Surgical assessment of pathologic N disease was obtained for 851 patients with M0 disease. Among these patients, 62% had pN0, 7% had pN1, 30% had pN2, and 1% had pN3. The median survivals for pN0, pN1, and pN2 were 24.0, 16.9, and 17.4 months, respectively. pN3 was excluded secondary to low numbers. Similar to the T descriptor with surgical confirmation, the final pathologic N stage was higher than the clinical N stage in 33% of patients, whereas it was lower in only 6% of the patients (**Fig. 3**).

The method and extent of nodal sampling were not standardized and varied significantly between institutions, therefore exploratory analyses were performed but not incorporated into the staging system. Exploratory analysis queried whether the number and extent of nodal stations influenced survival.[18] First, given that no difference in OS was noted between pN1 and pN2, these categories were analyzed together (pN+), which revealed a significantly worse survival compared with pN0. In addition, no differences were noted between patients with pN1 or pN2 single-station versus multiple-station disease. To examine the extent of disease, pN2 was

compared with pN1 and pN2 combined, which revealed that patients with combined disease (14 months) had significantly worse survival than pN2 only (19 months). Other analyses were performed for the total number of nodes, the lymph node ratios, and distribution. No differences were observed; however, the number of patients with sufficient data for these comparisons was low. Collectively, these findings suggest that anatomic location of nodal metastasis is less important than the cumulative extent of nodal involvement. For this reason, the staging classification was revised such that N1 denotes ipsilateral intrathoracic nodal metastasis and N2 denotes contralateral or any supraclavicular nodal metastasis.

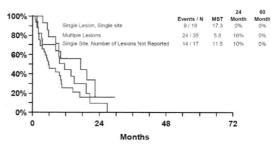

Fig. 4. OS of patients with single or multiple metastatic (M1) lesions from malignant pleural mesothelioma. M0, no distant metastasis; M1, distant metastasis present. (*From* Rusch VW, Chansky K, Kindler HL, et al. The IASLC Mesothelioma Staging Project: proposals for the M descriptors and for revision of the TNM staging groupings in the forthcoming eighth edition of the TNM Classification for Mesothelioma. J Thorac Oncol. 2016;11(12):2115; with permission.)

Similar to the T descriptor, whether tumor thickness predicted nodal metastasis was explored with 3 levels (upper, middle, and lower) of cut points based on maximal thickness.[18] Measurements of tumor thickness and complete N disease were available for 472 patients. With the same cut point of 5.1 mm that was generated for the T descriptor, the risks of nodal metastases less than and greater than that thickness were 14% and 38%. These findings were exploratory and require further investigation with more sophisticated technology before incorporation into the staging classifications.

Several weaknesses of nodal staging remain despite the improvements in this revision. First, the incidence of nodal metastasis depends on the extent of nodal sampling, which varies between surgeons, institutions, and the type of resection performed. Second, for patients who were staged both clinically and pathologically, clinical nodal staging did not accurately predict

Table 4
The tumor, node, metastasis staging for malignant pleural mesothelioma

Stage	Definition
Primary Tumor (T)	
TX	Primary tumor cannot be assessed
T0	No evidence of primary tumor
T1	Tumor limited to the ipsilateral parietal ± visceral ± mediastinal ± diaphragmatic pleura
T2	Tumor involving each of the ipsilateral pleural surfaces (parietal, mediastinal, diaphragmatic, and visceral pleura) with at least 1 of the following features: • Involvement of diaphragmatic muscle • Extension of tumor from visceral pleura into the underlying pulmonary parenchyma
T3	Describes locally advanced but potentially resectable tumor. Tumor involving all of the ipsilateral pleural surfaces (parietal, mediastinal, diaphragmatic, and visceral pleura) with at least 1 of the following features: • Involvement of the endothoracic fascia • Extension into the mediastinal fat • Solitary, completely resectable focus of tumor extending into the soft tissues of the chest wall • Nontransmural involvement of the pericardium
T4	Describes locally advanced technically unresectable tumor. Tumor involving all of the ipsilateral pleural surfaces (parietal, mediastinal, diaphragmatic, and visceral pleura) with at least 1 of the following features: • Diffuse extension or multifocal masses of tumor in the chest wall, with or without associated rib destruction • Direct transdiaphragmatic extension of tumor to the peritoneum • Direct extension of tumor to the contralateral pleura • Direct extension of tumor to mediastinal organs • Direct extension of tumor into the spine • Tumor extending through to the internal surface of the pericardium with or without a pericardial effusion, or tumor involving the myocardium
Regional Lymph Nodes (N)	
NX	Regional lymph nodes cannot be assessed
N0	No regional lymph node metastases
N1	Metastases in the ipsilateral bronchopulmonary, hilar, or mediastinal (including the internal mammary, peridiaphragmatic, pericardial fat pad, or intercostal lymph nodes) lymph nodes
N2	Metastases in the contralateral mediastinal, ipsilateral, or contralateral supraclavicular lymph nodes
Distant Metastasis (M)	
M0	No distant metastasis
M1	Distant metastasis present

From Rusch VW, Chansky K, Kindler HL, et al. The IASLC Mesothelioma Staging Project: proposals for the M descriptors and for revision of the TNM staging groupings in the forthcoming eighth edition of the TNM Classification for Mesothelioma. J Thorac Oncol. 2016;11(12):2117; with permission.

pathologic status.[4] The investigators did recommend use of invasive pretreatment nodal sampling to improve accuracy of clinical nodal staging.

M Descriptors for Malignant Pleural Mesothelioma

In the eighth edition of the TNM classifications for pleural mesothelioma, M0 and M1 denote absence and presence of distant metastases, respectively.[18] No changes were recommended to the M descriptor in the 2016 revision of MPM staging; however, the M descriptor was validated based on sufficient differences in OS between clinical M0 and M1. Importantly, the OS of patients with cM1 disease was compared with cM0 with locally advanced disease (T4 or N3) and showed a survival difference, which provided the rationale for including only cM1 in the stage IV group. The median OSs for cM1 versus T3 or N3 patients were 9.7 months versus 13.4 months, respectively. These data were generated from 2414 analyzable cases, although only 84 had cM1 disease.

Evaluation of the prognosis based on the location and number of metastatic sites was limited to exploratory analysis given the small group of 84 patients. In addition, only 70 patients had data regarding the site of disease. The differences in OS between patients with a single sites versus multiple sites suggested that patients with a single site have a better prognosis (**Fig. 4**). Additional data may confirm these findings and prompt revision to the M descriptor in the future.

Tumor, Node, Metastasis Staging for Malignant Pleural Mesothelioma

The staging for MPM based on the revised eighth edition of the TNM classifications includes T1N0M0 as stage IA, T2-3N0M0 as stage IB, T1-2N1M0 as stage II, T3N1M0 as stage IIIA, T1-2N2M0 and T4N0-2M0 as stage IIIB, and M1 as stage IV (**Table 4**).[18] These staging categories represent a substantial revision for the UICC/AJCC staging system of robust survival data among 3519 submitted cases. The OSs based on these stages are presented in **Fig. 5**.

Although this system is developed from an international, multi-institutional cohort study, the committee for IMIG and IASLC/SPFC stress the continued need for data collection and additional revisions for future revisions. At present, the staging project continues with the goal to develop recommendations for the ninth edition of the TNM. The study population for the ongoing project includes patients with newly diagnosed MPM. The data elements are more extensive than the prior databases and will include patient characteristics, laboratory

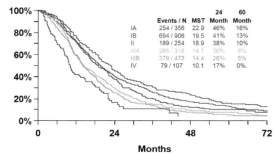

Fig. 5. OS of patients with malignant pleural mesothelioma based on the best staging for the eighth edition of the staging system. (*From* Rusch VW, Chansky K, Kindler HL, et al. The IASLC Mesothelioma Staging Project: proposals for the M descriptors and for revision of the TNM staging groupings in the forthcoming eighth edition of the TNM Classification for Mesothelioma. J Thorac Oncol. 2016;11(12):2116; with permission.)

values, pulmonary function tests, and standard uptake values from PET imaging to obtain pretreatment clinical TNM data. Pathologic TNM data will be obtained for surgically managed patients. The surgical data specifically will include data on extension into other structures for refinement of the T stage, nodal station involvement based on the IASLC 2009 nodal map for N stage refinements, and details for the M descriptor. Survival data will be obtained as expected. Collaborating institutions will receive data element lists to help standardize processes for collecting this information.

SUMMARY

MPM is a rare and deadly cancer of the thoracic serous membranes. The staging of this disease is challenging secondary to the low incidence and poor survival. At least 5 staging systems were proposed before 1990, before the first consensus system in 1994 by the IASLC. This system used TNM designations and borrowed heavily from parenchymal lung cancer descriptors. The IASLC formed a database to prospectively collect complete patient data and obtained more than 3000 cases from 1995 to 2013. In 2016, evidence-based revisions to the 1994 IASLC staging classification were released. Clinical staging now is based on findings from patients with MPM rather than lung cancer. However, several limitations still exist; therefore, ongoing efforts are underway at IASLC to improve staging with the next edition.

CLINICS CARE POINTS

- In 1995, IASLC published a universal TNM system for staging MPM based partially on lung cancer staging paradigms.

- In 2016, IASLC published revisions to the TNM system based on MPM cases collected from 1995 to 2013.
- Given the poor discrimination between T1a and T1b on both clinical and pathologic staging, a single T1 stage was adopted, and T1a and T1b were eliminated.
- The pathologic T stage was higher in 56% of clinical T1 patients, 54% of clinical T2 patients, and 39% of clinical T3 patients. Only 4% were assigned a lower pathologic stage than the clinical stage.
- The nodal staging classification was revised such that N1 denotes ipsilateral intrathoracic nodal metastasis and N2 denotes contralateral or any supraclavicular nodal metastasis. The distinction of N1 and N2 based on intraparenchymal versus mediastinal lymph nodes, similar to lung cancer staging, was eliminated. The N3 descriptor was removed.
- The pathologic N stage was higher than the clinical N stage in 33% of patients, whereas it was lower in only 6% of patients.
- No changes were recommended to the M descriptor, which was validated based on sufficient differences in OS between clinical cM0 and cM1.
- The revised eighth edition of the TNM classifications include T1N0M0 as stage IA, T2-3N0M0 as stage IB, T1-2N1M0 as stage II, T3N1M0 as stage IIIA, T1-2N2M0 and T4N0-2M0 as stage IIIB, and M1 as stage IV.
- Ongoing international efforts are underway to revise the current staging system with recommendations for the ninth edition of the TNM.

DISCLOSURE

The authors have nothing to disclose.

REFERENCES

1. Corson JM. Pathology of diffuse malignant pleural mesothelioma. Semin Thorac Cardiovasc Surg 1997;9(4):347–55.
2. Wagner JC, Sleggs CA, Marchand P. Diffuse pleural mesothelioma and asbestos exposure in the North Western Cape Province. Br J Ind Med 1960;17:260–71.
3. Attanoos RL, Gibbs AR. Pathology of malignant mesothelioma. Histopathology 1997;30(5):403–18.
4. Husain AN, et al. Guidelines for pathologic diagnosis of malignant mesothelioma: 2012 update of the consensus statement from the International Mesothelioma Interest Group. Arch Pathol Lab Med 2013;137(5):647–67.
5. Hammar SP, et al. Mucin-positive epithelial mesotheliomas: a histochemical, immunohistochemical, and ultrastructural comparison with mucin-producing pulmonary adenocarcinomas. Ultrastruct Pathol 1996;20(4):293–325.
6. Attanoos RL, Gibbs AR. 'Pseudomesotheliomatous' carcinomas of the pleura: a 10-year analysis of cases from the Environmental Lung Disease Research Group, Cardiff. Histopathology 2003;43(5):444–52.
7. Crotty EJ, et al. Epithelioid hemangioendothelioma of the pleura: clinical and radiologic features. AJR Am J Roentgenol 2000;175(6):1545–9.
8. Rusch VW. A proposed new international TNM staging system for malignant pleural mesothelioma. From the International Mesothelioma Interest Group. Chest 1995;108(4):1122–8.
9. Pass H, et al. The IASLC mesothelioma staging project: improving staging of a rare disease through international participation. J Thorac Oncol 2016;11(12):2082–8.
10. Tammilehto L, et al. Evaluation of the clinical TNM staging system for malignant pleural mesothelioma: an assessment in 88 patients. Lung Cancer 1995;12(1–2):25–34.
11. Butchart EG, et al. Pleuropneumonectomy in the management of diffuse malignant mesothelioma of the pleura. Experience with 29 patients. Thorax 1976;31(1):15–24.
12. Sugarbaker DJ, et al. Node status has prognostic significance in the multimodality therapy of diffuse, malignant mesothelioma. J Clin Oncol 1993;11(6):1172–8.
13. Chahinian AP, et al. Diffuse malignant mesothelioma. Prospective evaluation of 69 patients. Ann Intern Med 1982;96(6 Pt 1):746–55.
14. Pass HI, et al. Preoperative tumor volume is associated with outcome in malignant pleural mesothelioma. J Thorac Cardiovasc Surg 1998;115(2):310–7 [discussion: 317–8].
15. Rusch VW, Venkatraman E. The importance of surgical staging in the treatment of malignant pleural mesothelioma. J Thorac Cardiovasc Surg 1996;111(4):815–25 [discussion: 825–6].
16. Rusch VW, et al. Initial analysis of the international association for the study of lung cancer mesothelioma database. J Thorac Oncol 2012;7(11):1631–9.
17. Nowak AK, et al. The IASLC mesothelioma staging project: proposals for revisions of the T descriptors in the forthcoming eighth edition of the TNM classification for pleural mesothelioma. J Thorac Oncol 2016;11(12):2089–99.
18. Rusch VW, et al. The IASLC mesothelioma staging project: proposals for the M descriptors and for revision of the TNM Stage Groupings in the Forthcoming (Eighth) Edition of the TNM classification for mesothelioma. J Thorac Oncol 2016;11(12):2112–9.

Preoperative Identification of Benefit from Surgery for Malignant Pleural Mesothelioma

Isabelle Opitz, MD*, Katarzyna Furrer, MD

KEYWORDS

- Malignant pleural mesothelioma • Surgery • Survival • Prognostic factors

KEY POINTS

- Patients with malignant pleural mesothelioma have a poor prognosis.
- In current guidelines, surgery is the recommended option in selected patients with early-stage disease as part of a multimodal approach.
- Preoperative identification of factors associated with improved outcome is crucial for decision-making.
- The available literature for prognostic factors and scores for treatment allocation for surgery are presented.

INTRODUCTION

Malignant pleural mesothelioma (MPM) is a rare, aggressive, and devastating disease of the thoracic cavity associated with asbestos exposure. In recent years, MPM incidence has been rising and, although the use of asbestos has been prohibited in 55 countries, it is not expected to decrease until 2030.[1,2] A report from the International Agency for Research on Cancer indicates that the disease burden is still substantial, with 30,443 cases of malignant mesothelioma and 25,576 deaths worldwide according to GLOBO-CAN 2018 statistics.[3,4] The treatment options are restricted by the poor prognosis and short life expectancy of 8 to 15 months[5] from diagnosis. Surgery is part of the most effective multimodality treatment in prolonging survival and is a possible option for patients with a good prognosis in high-volume experienced centers.[3]

Selection criteria for surgery and identification of the appropriate candidate are crucial, and it is strongly recommended that a maximal surgical cytoreduction should be performed.[6] Maximal surgical cytoreduction as a single-modality treatment is generally insufficient; additional antineoplastic treatment (chemotherapy and/or radiation therapy) should be administered.[6] It is recommended that any treatment decision should be made with multidisciplinary input involving thoracic surgeons, pulmonologists, medical and radiation oncologists, radiologists, and pathologists to find the best therapeutic options for each individual patient.[6]

To provide recommendation for identification of benefit from surgery, many factors have to be taken into account: selection of candidates for surgery by clinical predicators and pathology with summary of the different predictor scores, as well as availability and access to different treatment approaches. This article summarizes these prognostic factors.

CLINICAL AND RADIOLOGIC PREOPERATIVE PROGNOSTIC FACTORS

Research focused on identification of clinical selection criteria for surgery in a multimodality

Department of Thoracic Surgery, University Hospital Zurich, Raemistrasse 100, Zurich 8091, Switzerland
* Corresponding author.
E-mail address: Isabelle.schmitt-opitz@usz.ch

Thorac Surg Clin 30 (2020) 435–449
https://doi.org/10.1016/j.thorsurg.2020.08.003
1547-4127/20/

therapy approach was initiated in 1976, when Butchart and colleagues[7] in Newcastle (UK) described the importance of precise patient selection for surgery. Butchart was one of the pioneers in mesothelioma surgery and concluded that death could have been prevented by better case selection, alteration in surgical technique, and better postoperative management.[7]

The unpredictable biological behavior of mesothelioma, the lack of correlation between clinical and pathologic staging, and patients' individual risk factors make the best treatment allocation difficult for an individual patient.

In general, specific considerations such as clinical factors (patients' demographics, performance status, specific prognostic markers in blood[8–13] and pleural effusion,[14] serologic markers of inflammation[15] and activated immune response,[16,17] cardiac[18] and pulmonary assessments,[19] radiologic staging, and tumor response to neoadjuvant chemotherapy) and pathologic factors (histology, genetic background, and molecular biomarkers), together with prognostic scores to select the patients for curative MPM surgery, are discussed in this article.

Historically, Butchart and colleagues[7] divided their cohort of 29 patients in 1976 into "fit" and "unfit" for surgery and categorized them additionally into "above 60 years" or "below 60 years" of age. In general, age and, in early publications, white race were predictors for cancer-directed surgery,[20] and advanced age was frequently mentioned as a significant factor associated with poor survival in previous reports.[21–24] With changing demographics, age is currently a less stringent exclusion criterion for surgery; however, in the literature the age limit for favorable outcome varies from younger than 45 years[25] to younger than 70 years[6] (overall survival [OS] 19.8 vs 11.7 months; $P<.001$, multivariate analysis)[26] as an independent prognostic factor, and surgery was associated with improved survival in patients aged ≥70 years but not in those aged ≥80 years in a Cox proportional hazards survival model published by Yang and colleagues.[23] Consistent with these results, the Beijing group of Zhuo and colleagues[27] used the recent SEER (Surveillance, Epidemiology, and End Results) database to produce a nomogram showing that the mortality risk increases strongly with increasing age in patients older than 70 years. Thus, surgery on patients older than 70 years must be very carefully decided upon because it may not translate into a survival benefit.[27] Another prognosticator of outcome and survival after surgery for MPM is gender. Female gender was associated with improved survival[21,28] (OS 12.0 vs 9.9 months, $P<.001$;[29] and 22 [95%

confidence interval (CI)] 18–30] vs 14 months [95% CI 13–16][25]). Male gender (hazard ratio [HR] 1.486, 95% CI 1.241–1.77[25]) was independently associated with reduced OS (all $P<.05$).[27] Circulating estrogen, present in young but not older women, and the expression of the estrogen receptor β, have been suggested to play a role in the survival difference between genders.[30,31] In one of the first studies by Curran and colleagues[10] the combination of poor performance status Eastern Cooperative Oncology Group (ECOG) status 1 or 2, high white blood cell (WBC) count (>8.3 × 10⁹/L), and male gender were in general associated with poor prognosis,[32,33] whereas ECOG status 0 (27.4 vs 9.7 months; $P = .015$) was a preoperative factor predicting benefit for surgery and survival.[29] Analyses of large datasets defined negative prognostic factors such as poor performance status (PS), low hemoglobin (Hb) count, male gender, high platelet count, high lactate dehydrogenase (LDH) level, and high WBC count.[12] Neutrophil-to-lymphocyte ratio (NLR) less than 5 (11.9 vs 7.5 months; $P<.001$), platelet count less than 400 G/L (11.5 vs 7.2 months; $P<.001$) and normal Hb (16.4 vs 8.8 months; $P<.001$) are factors predicting benefit for MPM surgery and long-term survival.[29,34] C-reactive protein (CRP) is a typical inflammation-related independent prognostic biomarker (HR 2.07, 95% CI 1.23–3.46; $P = .01$), and patients with increased levels in blood had shorter OS in comparison with normal CRP (CRP ≥1 mg/dL: HR 2.81, 95% CI 1.82–4.33; $P<.001$).[16] Furthermore, increased CRP in pleural effusion[35] was associated with worse outcome (CRP ≥3.8 mg/dL: HR 2.288, CI 1.505–3.478; $P<.001$).[36]

Other hematologic markers associated with diagnosis and prognosis (discussed in detail in Harvey I. Pass and colleagues' article, "Mesothelioma Biomarkers: Discovery in Search of Validation," in this issue) include soluble mesothelin-related proteins, osteopontin, Fibulin-3, high-mobility group box 1 (HMGB1), lymphocyte-to-monocyte ratio (LMR), NLR, and platelet-to-lymphocyte ratio (PLR).[37,38] HMGB1, a damage-associated molecular pattern protein released by necrotic cells, has diagnostic and prognostic value,[39,40] with an inverse association between HMGB1 serum levels and survival at a cutoff value of 9 ng/mL. Lastly, the most promising hematologic marker is the peripheral blood marker LMR, given its proven correlation with survival. Yamagishi and colleagues[41] showed that patients with LMR serum level greater than 2.74 had longer OS of 14 months in comparison with 5 months at a lower level.

Current guidelines of the British Thoracic Society (BTS) recommend the use of specific factors to determine prognosis at baseline and timing of treatment.[42] These comprise demographic factors (age, gender, race), disease features (histologic subtype and grade, site of disease, disease stage using various staging systems), ECOG PS or Karnofski performance score, symptoms (chest pain, weight loss), total WBC count, platelet count, NLR, PLR, CRP level, and blood test markers such as Hb level, Hb difference from a population ideal value (160 g/L in men, 140 g/L in women), and serum albumin (all grade D).[42]

Concerning the application of the of the non–tissue-based biomarkers for diagnosis, predicting outcome, or monitoring tumor response, the current American Society of Clinical Oncology (ASCO) guidelines state that these markers are under evaluation and at this time do not have the sensitivity or specificity to predict outcome or monitor tumor response, and are therefore not recommended (Type of recommendation: evidence based; Evidence quality: intermediate; Strength of recommendation: moderate).[6]

The selection process based on radiologic features to decide which patients are eligible for surgery is challenging and requires expertise and interdisciplinary collaboration. According to current ASCO guidelines, patients with transdiaphragmatic disease and multifocal chest wall invasion (ie, all features that exclude patients from macroscopic complete resection [MCR]) should undergo neoadjuvant treatment before consideration of maximal surgical cytoreduction.[6] These staging questions should be addressed by the following investigations: computed tomography (CT) scan with intravenous (IV) contrast (chest and upper abdomen) and [18F]fluorodeoxyflucose PET/CT (18F-FDG PET/CT) scan (Type of recommendation: evidence based; Evidence quality: intermediate; Strength of recommendation: strong) or MRI, particularly with IV contrast (Type of recommendation: evidence based; Evidence quality: intermediate; Strength of recommendation: moderate), as recommended by ASCO guidelines.[6]

In accordance with BTS guidelines, concerning imaging modalities for diagnosing and staging, CT scan of thorax with IV contrast is recommended for the initial imaging modality as well as PET/CT to exclude distant metastases—but not for aiding diagnosis in patients who have had prior talc pleurodesis and with caution in populations with a high prevalence of tuberculosis—in addition to MRI for patients in whom differentiating T stage will change management (all grade D).[42] In general, the radiologic staging often has a poor correlation with pathologic staging.[43] Additional radiologic assessments with functional imaging techniques using MRI, such as diffusion-weighted imaging (DWI) and dynamic contrast-enhanced (DCE) MRI with 18F-FDG PET/CT, can rule out chest wall infiltration, transdiaphragmatic infiltration, nodal involvement, or occult metastasis at the same time.[44,45]

Although staging algorithms for MPM are discussed in detail in R. Taylor Ripley's article, "Extended Pleurectomy and Decortication for Malignant Pleural Mesothelioma," in this issue, a word about exclusion of patients from surgery based on clinical stage is timely. Overall, the decision to undergo surgery should still be made on an individual basis.

Traditionally, TNM stage is the classic prognosticator for cancer treatment. Both parameters—T stage and N stage—combined with epithelial histology, female gender, and adjuvant therapy are the traditionally identified prognostic factors in patients with MPM[46]; however, nowadays the discrimination between T2 and T3 (infiltration of chest wall) is almost impossible. Moreover, there are no precise selection criteria based on T factors alone.[47–49] The current American Joint Committee on Cancer/Union for International Cancer Control classification[50] mentions difficulties in applying it to clinical staging with respect to both T and N parameters, resulting in imprecise predicted prognosis; moreover, as strongly recommended in ASCO guidelines, clinicians should recognize that in patients with clinical stage I/II disease, upstaging may occur at surgery.[6] In the last proposals for revision of the T descriptors, survival correlated with pleural thickness. Pleural thickness showed an increase at higher T stages and was significantly associated with node positivity and overall stage. Based on these findings and data from the seventh edition of T categories and overall stage, survival showed a median of 23.4 months for the lowest tumor thickness (<16.0 mm) vs 13.2 months for the highest tumor thickness (>50.0 mm).[51] Nevertheless, further investigations as to whether tumor thickness should be included in future staging systems are necessary. Tumor stages I to III are included if deemed technically resectable, with most of the patients treated within clinical trial protocols. Decisions leading to surgery are made individually, and even localized chest wall infiltration is accepted if chest wall resection seems feasible and reasonable at only one level.

In this regard, another important prognosticator is the status of mediastinal lymph node involvement (N factor), which is a poor prognostic factor for MPM as mentioned in several studies 2 decades ago.[46,52,53] Mediastinal staging is performed with PET/CT, EBUS/FNA (endobrachial ultrasound elastography/fine-needle aspiration), or mediastinoscopy to exclude N3 disease.[54] Patients with histologically confirmed contralateral mediastinal or supraclavicular lymph node involvement should undergo neoadjuvant treatment before consideration of maximal surgical cytoreduction according to recent ASCO guidelines.[6] The proposal for current eighth edition of the International Association for the Study of Lung Cancer Mesothelioma Staging Project showed that for clinically staged tumors there was no difference between cN0, cN1, or cN2 (cN1 vs cN0: HR 1.06, $P = .77$ and cN2 vs cN1: HR 1.04, $P = .85$), and patients with pN1 or pN2 tumors had shorter survival than those with pN0 tumors (HR 1.51, $P<.0001$), but no survival difference was observed between those with pN1 and pN2 tumors (HR 0.99, $P = .99$). Patients with concurrent pN1/pN2 nodal involvement had poorer survival than those with pN2 tumors alone (HR 1.60, $P = .007$) or pN0 tumors (HR 1.62, $P<.0001$).[55] Occult nodal disease detected during resection for cN0 MPM correlate with higher hazard of mortality ($P = .005$)[56] and poorer prognosis with similar survival as cN+ cases. These data underline the importance of routine preoperative pathologic nodal assessment for potentially resectable MPM and that the number of involved lymph nodes (rather than current location-based classification) is associated with OS and may provide more robust prognostic stratification for future TNM staging.[56]

In conclusion, this means that nodal involvement seems to be of prognostic importance, although the location in the mediastinum needs to be interpreted differently from lung cancer. Therefore, the N-descriptor was revised for the eighth TNM classification to more MPM-specific N-categories in comparison with the seventh edition, where the median survival for cN0 patients was 19 months vs 17.6 and 16.2 months for cN1 and cN2 patients, respectively, without statistical significance.[55] Surgery alone for patients with positive ipsilateral mediastinal lymph nodes is not appropriate, and a multimodality approach, particularly as part of a clinical trial, should be considered.[6]

Selecting MPM patients for surgery based on response to chemotherapy or other treatments as a marker for biological behaviors is another opportunity. However, radiologic assessment of tumor response to treatment using standard RECIST (Response Evaluation Criteria in Solid Tumors) criteria that require bidimensional measurements is not practical and often difficult in monitoring of mesothelioma,[57] because the morphology and growth pattern of mesothelioma differs substantively from that of other solid tumors.[58] Based on restaging imaging by contrast-enhanced CT or ^{18}F-FDG PET/CT imaging after induction chemotherapy and assessment of modified RECIST (mRECIST) criteria,[59] patients are classified as progressive disease, stable disease, or partial response, and whether they are potentially resectable or not. This method requires acquisition of up to 6 measurements of tumor thickness, each at least 1 cm in extent, perpendicular to the chest wall or mediastinum[59,60] with no more than 2 measurement sites on each of 3 separate CT sections separated axially by at least 1 cm,[59] involving a multistage process with variability between observers at each of these steps.[61] Consequently, this should be performed by a radiologist familiar with mRECIST for MPM.[62] Complete or partial radiologic response is associated with improved median survival of 26.0 vs 13.9 months for patients with stable disease or progressive disease ($P = .05$).[63] However, progressive disease alone is not an exclusion criterion per se for surgery as long as MCR is still feasible (**Fig. 1** and Opitz and colleagues, unpublished data).

For a more accurate evaluation of resectability in terms of tumor load, tumor volume measured before and after induction treatment is an attractive parameter. Conventional quantitative measurement of the tumor volume (**Fig. 2**)[47] and newly deep convolutional neural network (CNN)-automated volumetric segmentation of MPM tumor on CT scans[64] has been a field of interest for prognostic evaluation of tumor staging[65] and response with reduction in tumor volume on CT[66] or MRI[67] after neoadjuvant treatment,[47,68,69] as well as prediction of survival.[66] Furthermore, already observed increasing tumor volume and decreasing lung volume during neoadjuvant chemotherapy are both significantly and independently associated with poor prognosis.[70]

As described first in 1998 by Pass and colleagues,[71] preoperatively assessed tumor volume can predict OS and progression-free survival (PFS) as well as postoperative stage. Large volumes are associated with nodal spread as well as postresection residual tumor burden and may predict the outcome.[47,65,71,72] In another study, Gill and colleagues[73] showed poorer OS if the tumor volume was greater than 500 cm^3, confirmed by Rusch and colleagues,[65] who reported that tumor volumes of 91.2, 245.3, and 511.3 cm^3 were associated with a median OS of 37, 18, and 8 months, respectively.

Radiomic biomarkers had a stronger prognostic value compared with tumor volume alone. The

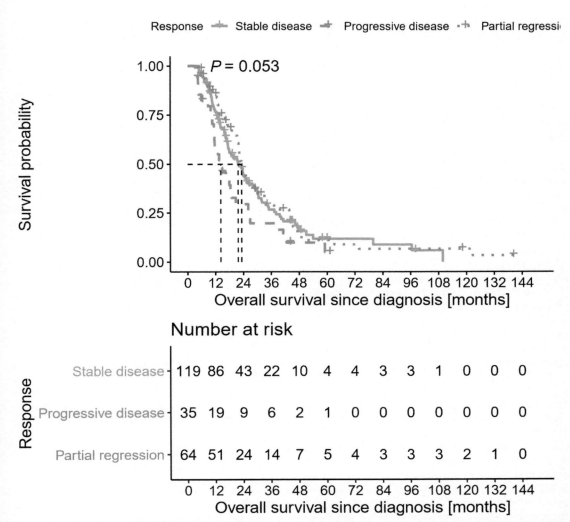

Fig. 1. Intention to treat (ITT) by response defined according to mRECIST criteria by independent observers (T.F., C.Z., D.-L.N.)[59] in N = 218 patients before and after induction as was the tumor volume, which was assessed by the help of semiautomated dedicated software as described previously.[47] Partial regression does not seem more beneficial compared with stable disease when considering survival times (HR, 0.9067194; CI, [0.6404001, 1.2837914]; P = .58). However, a progressive disease response is associated with a significantly higher risk of dying compared with a stable disease response (HR, 1.5496089; CI, [1.0230936, 2.347085]; P = .04).

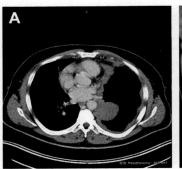 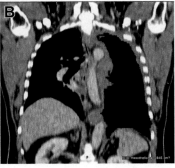

Fig. 2. Volumetry of malignant pleural mesothelioma. (*A,B*) The marked tumor (*green*) on a single CT slice.[47]

authors evaluated radiomic features (shape, intensity, texture [relation of an individual pixel to its neighborhood], and wavelet decomposition), a promising methodology for quantitative analysis and description of radiologic images using advanced mathematics and statistics in CT images, and a prognostic model for OS in MPM patients was developed based on these CT image characteristics.[74] Two wavelet features were prognostic for OS in multivariable Cox regression (concordance index: 0.74; $P = .002$). Both features separated the patients into 2 groups with a significantly different OS ($P = .0006$) and a significantly different PFS ($P = .003$).[69]

MRI offers higher contrast resolution than CT and is therefore potentially more appropriate for volumetric analyses.[75] Tumor volumes ($\geq$300 mL) had significantly poorer median OS (multivariable Cox proportional hazards model, HR 2.114 [1.046–4.270], $P = .037$).[69] However, the observed difference in median OS with tumor volume increased when analysis was restricted to patients with epithelioid histology and further increased when epithelioid cases with nodal or metastatic disease were excluded.[69]

Other functional imaging techniques using DWI and DCE MRI have the potential to act as a quantitative method of assessing tumor response to treatment.[57] These techniques are reflective of the underlying tumor pathophysiology, such as tissue cellularity and microvessel density.[57] In the analysis of preoperative prediction of unresectability in MPM, Burt and colleagues[76] proposed a novel metric of thoracic cage volume, calculated by preoperative chest CT scan, and determined associations between preoperative variables and diffuse chest wall invasion (DCWI) and contraction of thoracic cage volume in patients scheduled for MCR. Decreased ipsilateral thoracic cage volume demonstrated the strongest association with unresectability by DCWI ($P = .009$), with greater than 5% decrease representing the optimal cutoff ($P = .014$; area under the curve, 0.67). Preoperative identification of DCWI can avoid unnecessary thoracotomy and accelerate initiation of nonsurgical therapy.[76] Other variables associated with DCWI included chest pain requiring opioids ($P = .028$), pleurodesis ($P = .036$), decreased forced vital capacity (FVC) ($P = .023$), decreased ipsilateral lung perfusion ($P = .007$), and chest wall invasion ($P = .035$).[76]

Another potential selection tool for surgery or supportive factor in the decision-making process is the prognostic significance of maximum standardized uptake value (SUV_{max}) as assessed by ^{18}F-FDG PET/CT, which measures tumor activity and functional tumor volume to indicate patient prognosis[77] and is the focus of continued research and clinical investigation.[69] However, PET should be interpreted with caution in patients after talc pleurodesis.[6] Recently, Lim and colleagues[78] proposed SUV_{max} as an independent prognostic factor in all patients ($P = .003$), especially those with the epithelioid subtype associated with OS ($P = .012$), but not in those with a nonepithelioid subtype.

Finally, an important factor is the patients' individual expectation of postoperative quality of life (QoL). Despite not unsubstantially reduced overall QoL regarding ability to perform everyday activities that reflect physical, psychological, and social well-being, and patient satisfaction with levels of functioning and control of the disease after surgery, some of these studies demonstrate a tendency for better QoL (physical function, social function, and global health were better at follow-up) after lung-sparing surgery[79] after 6 and 12 months,[80] whereas other indicators such as pain and cough were similar.[79] This might be related to the fact that with decortication of entrapped lungs, lung function and, therefore, QoL can improve. Predicted postoperative FEV_1 (forced expiratory volume in 1 s) and FVC were reported in one study only and were higher at follow-up for pleurectomy/decortication (P/D) compared with extrapleural pneumonectomy (EPP).[81]

Pathologic Subtypes, and Genetic and Molecular Factors

Benefit from surgery and survival for MPM is significantly affected by tumor histology. The histologic subtypes of MPM with epithelioid, sarcomatoid, and biphasic type have clear prognostic significance,[6] which might help in selecting patients for intensive multimodal treatment approaches and in identifying whether patients are eligible for surgery. The biphasic subtype showed poor prognosis compared with the epithelioid subtype, whereas prognosis of the sarcomatoid subtype was worst in a recently published analysis of the SEER database[27] and consistent with previous studies and guidelines.[6,8,10,29,52,53,82–84] Meyerhoff and colleagues[24] reported that most common epithelioid histology is related to better survival compared with biphasic or sarcomatoid histology (19 vs 12 vs 4 months in the sarcomatoid group [$P<.01$]) and in multivariate analysis, surgery was associated with improved survival in the epithelioid group (HR 0.72, $P<.01$) but not in biphasic (HR 0.73, $P = .19$) and sarcomatoid (HR 0.79, $P = .18$) groups regardless of type of surgical resection.

According to the World Health Organization 2015 classification[83,85] of epithelioid MPM, histologic subtypes of predominantly microcystic/tubulopapillary pattern were associated with longer OS than the solid/trabecular subtype (732 vs 397 days, P = .0013), whereas the pleomorphic subtype had the shortest OS (173 days).[86] The solid/trabecular variants showed a significant association with a high nuclear grade and mitosis-necrosis score as an independent prognostic factor.[86] In a group of patients who received multimodal treatment, those with tubulopapillary/microcystic pattern MPMs showed a tendency toward better OS than those with solid/trabecular pattern tumors (HR 2.29, 95% CI 0.95–5.12; P = .066).[86]

Another current subject of further investigation is grading, whereby well or moderately differentiated subtypes resulted in better prognoses than poorly differentiated or undifferentiated subtypes,[27] suggesting that nuclear atypia and mitotic count are independent preoperative prognostic markers for MPM.[83]

In conclusion, according to ASCO guidelines surgery is not recommended in patients with sarcomatoid MPM[6]; however, in carefully selected cases biphasic or sarcomatoid subtype with negative mediastinal lymph node status is not obliged to be excluded from surgery because this can be the only option for these patients, given their higher incidence of chemoresistance.[52,87,88] Therefore, the decision for or against surgery should not be based on a single factor such as histotype but rather a combination of various factors, given that there are certain subtypes of epithelioid MPM— biphasic or sarcomatoid histotypes—with proven long-term survival.[89,90]

Genetic predisposition, as explored in preclinical studies, is an important predictor of disease progression and survival (discussed in detail in Benjamin Wadowski and colleagues' article, "The Molecular Basis of Malignant Pleural Mesothelioma," in this issue). To date, it has not been included in the decision-making process for or against surgery. In brief, genetic prognosticators include chromosome alterations of cyclin-dependent kinase inhibitor 2A (CDKN2A) locus (9p21.3), homozygous p16 deletions (especially for sarcomatous type), and BRCA1-associated protein 1 (BAP1) mutations, all of which are associated with poor prognosis.[91–93]

In the following a few molecular prognostic factors, being a focus of the authors' research area, are briefly discussed, though not in depth because this is the topic of Harvey I. Pass and colleagues' article, "Mesothelioma Biomarkers: Discovery in Search of Validation," in this issue. However, recommendations regarding the use of biomarkers from current guidelines[42] do not support biomarkers in isolation as a diagnostic (Grade B) or screening test (Grade C) or to predict treatment response or survival (Grade B) in MPM.

MicroRNAs (miRNAs) are small noncoding RNA molecules that regulate gene expression.[94,95] Kirschner and colleagues[96] established the miR-Score, consisting of 6 miRNAs (miR-21-5p, -23-3p, −30e-5p, 221-3p, -222-3p) for prediction of longer survival in positive patients.

MPM is characterized by complex chromosomal aberrations, including chromosome 10 losses and the tumor-suppressor gene phosphatase and tensin homolog deleted from chromosome 10 (PTEN) located on chromosome 10q23. The authors' group showed that median survival time was significantly longer in patients with PTEN expression (15.5 months: 95% CI 3.8, 27.2 vs 9.7 months: 95% CI 7.9, 11.7) independent of histologic subtype (P = .7).[97,98] Furthermore, Schramm and colleagues[99] demonstrated that low cytoplasmic periostin and high cytoplasmic PTEN are independent prognosticators of better OS.[99] In addition, the authors observed that a decrease in PTEN and an increase in p-mTOR (pathologic mammalian target of rapamycin) expression during induction chemotherapy were associated with shorter OS.[98] These investigations were recently confirmed by Kuroda and colleagues,[100] who moreover proposed that molecular-targeted treatment involving the mTOR signaling pathway might be used during multimodal therapy for MPM.

Another prognosticator is cytokine migration inhibitory factor (MIF) and its receptor CD74 together with calretinin in tissue microarray, which correlates with OS. CD74 (P<.001) but not MIF overexpression (P = .231) is an independent prognostic factor for prolonged OS.[101] Interestingly these positive results for CD74 were consistent with a previously published report that high expression of tumoral PTEN is an independent prognostic factor for prolonged OS in mesothelioma patients.[97] High expression of tumor cell calretinin correlated with the epithelioid histotype predicted longer OS (P<.001).[101] Thies and colleagues[102] correlated the neural crest stem cell marker nestin and the epithelial-mesenchymal transition marker periostin with histology and found that in platinum/pemetrexed-treated patients, nestin was higher in biphasic MPM compared with epithelioid MPM, Regarding expression of nestin in chemo-naïve biopsies (OS: 22 vs 17 months) and chemo-treated surgical specimens (OS: 18 vs 12 months), both nonepithelioid histology and high periostin level in biopsies (OS: 23 vs 15 months) were associated with poor prognosis. In the multivariate survival analysis, any nestin expression in chemo-naïve biopsies proved to be an independent prognosticator against histology.[102] Furthermore, Meerang and colleagues[103] discovered that low Merlin expression and high Survivin expression are also associated with a poorer prognosis. These investigators showed that cell proliferation marker Ki-67 and a high nuclear Survivin-labeling index in prechemotherapy and postchemotherapy tissues were associated with shorter freedom from recurrence.[98,103] Programmed death-ligand 1 (PD-L1) expression in tumor tissue was associated with a lower median survival of 6 vs 15.5 months compared with negative PD-L1, and positive PD-L1 expression ($\geq$1%) was independently correlated with poor prognosis (HR 2.02, 95% CI, 1.005–4.057, $P = .0484$).[104] Patients with PD-L1-positive tumors had shorter OS than patients with negative PD-L1 (HR 1.581, CI 1.043–2.396, $P = .031$).[36]

In summary, although all of these markers showed promising results, most have yet to be independently and prospectively validated, and for some of them controversial results from different studies concerning their prognostic impact need to be addressed.[38] So far, all these markers and their potential prognostic value have had no impact on patient selection in predicting outcome or monitoring tumor response,[6] but may be included in selection algorithms.

PROGNOSTIC SCORES

Because the use of a single factor to predict prognosis is not justified, with rather the synthesis of several factors leading to the decision for a curative operation, prognostic scores are of interest. Combining groups of prognostic variables originating from cohorts of patients and subsequent validation in different test cohorts[42] seems to be attractive for the identification of candidates for surgery. The European Organization for Research and Treatment of Cancer (EORTC) and the Cancer and Leukemia Group B (CALGB) developed a prognostic score and prognostic groups for better identification of patients receiving different chemotherapy regimens by analyzing the patients' pretreatment characteristics.[10,11]

The EORTC prognostic score[10] includes the ECOG PS, histologic subtype, gender, certainty of diagnosis (definitive vs possible), and defined good prognosis group (ECOG 0, epithelioid histology, female, definitive diagnosis, and WBC < 8.3 × 10⁹/L) and poor prognosis group (ECOG 1, nonepithelioid histology, male, possible diagnosis, and WBC > 8.3 × 10⁹/L). The CALGB

prognostic score is derived from 6 prognostic subgroups. Here poor ECOG PS, chest pain, dyspnea, platelet count greater than 400 G/L, weight loss, LDH level greater than 500 IU/L, pleural involvement, low Hb level, high WBC count, and age greater than 75 years predicted poor survival. Pleural involvement, LDH greater than 500 IU/L, poor PS, chest pain, PLT greater than 400,000/µL, nonepithelial histology, and age greater than 75 years predicted poor survival in multivariate analysis.[11] The subgroup with the best survival included patients with PS 0 and age less than 49 years, and patients with PS 0, age 49 years or older, and hemoglobin $\geq$14.6 g/L. The worst survival occurred for patients with PS 1/2 and WBC $\geq$ 15.6/µL.[11]

Edwards and colleagues[12] validated the effectiveness of the EORTC and CALGB scores as early as 20 years ago. Patients were stratified into low-risk and high-risk groups and correlated with the EORTC series with a median survival of 9.4 vs 10.8 months (low-risk group) and 3.8 vs 5.5 months (high-risk group), respectively.[12]. The EORTC score was recently evaluated by the Italian group of Sandri.[105] Multivariable analysis confirmed an independent prognostic value of EORTC score (HR 2.86, $P<.001$) as a reliable and valid instrument that may be implemented in daily practice.[105]

Furthermore, an Italian group explored predictors of long-term survival and defined a prognostic score in a multicenter analysis.[106] On multivariate analysis, younger age (OR 0.51, 95% CI 0.31–0.82), epithelioid histology (OR 7.07, 95% CI 1.56–31.93), no history of asbestos exposure (OR 3.13, 95% CI 1.13–8.66), and the ratio between metastatic and resected lymph nodes less than 22% (OR 4.12, 95% CI 1.68–10.12) were independent predictors of long-term survival. Long-term survival was defined as survival longer than 2 times the median OS (18 months) and stratified patients into 2 groups: 36 months (long-term survival group) and those surviving between 4 and 35 months (short-term survival group). The investigators created a scoring system (1–12 points) identifying patients for long-term survival with a score greater than 6 and predicting favorable overall, cancer-specific, and disease-free survival ($P<.0001$).[106]

Pass, Rusch, and colleagues[107,108] identified prognostically important and independent covariates for prediction of survival including stage, age, gender, histology (epithelioid vs nonepithelioid), and the type of surgical procedure (palliative vs curative), defined as "CORE" values, and analyzed their impact on OS: adjuvant therapy (yes: OS 18 months vs no: OS 10 months), smoking history (no: OS 16 months vs yes: OS

15 months), history of asbestos exposure (no: OS 17 months vs yes: OS 15 months), history of weight loss, defined as greater than 5% (OS 11 months) vs less than 5% (OS 17 months) in the previous 6 months, ECOG PS 0 (OS 22 months) and 1 (OS 16 months), chest pain (no: OS 19 months vs yes: OS 14 months); and dyspnea (no: OS 15 months vs yes: OS 17 months), Hb level (<14.6; OS 16 months vs >14.6 OS 20 months), platelet count (<400; OS 19 months vs >400 OS 12 months), WBC count (<15.5; OS 16 months vs >15.5 OS 8 months), and LDH level before surgery. In total, they defined 3 prognostic models with these covariates. Models 1 and 2 included the CORE variables. Model 1 additionally included adjuvant treatment, WBC, and platelet count, and model 2 consisted of the same covariates as model 1 but without a surgical staging, with Hb added as additional parameter. Model 3 showed only parameters available before surgery (histology, gender, age, WBC, Hb, and platelets) and therefore represented the potential surgery patient. The models per se were not analyzed according to their prognostic value; only their covariates were individually indicated as having prognostic significance and HR.[107,108]

The modified Glasgow Prognostic Score (mGPS) categorizes patients with cancer according to CRP and serum albumin.[15] This was found to be an independent predictor of OS in MPM (HR 2.6, 95% CI 1.6–4.2, $P<.001$)[15] and has not been further prospectively validated. Both mGPS and NLR were independent predictors of OS (HR 2.6 and 2.0, respectively).[15]

The LENT prognostic score was developed by Clive and colleagues[109] for predicting survival in patients presenting with malignant pleural effusion using LDH (>1500) IU/L, ECOG PS, NLR, and tumor type. Analysis of the area under the receiver-operating characteristic (ROC) curve revealed the LENT score to be superior at predicting survival compared with ECOG PS at 1 month ($P<.01$), 3 months ($P<.01$), and 6 months ($P<.01$).[109]

Another prognostic score using decision tree analysis was published by Brims and colleagues[110] who developed and validated a simple, clinically relevant model to discriminate patients at high and lower risk of death using routinely available variables from the time of diagnosis. The strongest predictive variable was the presence of weight loss. The group with the best survival at 18 months (86.7% alive, median survival 34.0 months, termed risk group 1) had no weight loss, an Hb level of >153 g/L, and a serum albumin level of >43 g/L. The group with the worst survival (0% alive, median survival 7.5 months, termed risk group 4d) had weight loss, a PS of 0 or 1, and sarcomatoid histologic characteristics.[110]

A Japanese group led by Doi[111] developed a new Novel Prognostic Risk Classification System.[111] Pathologic subtype, serum LDH, NLR ratio, and total lesion glycolysis (TLG) in ^{18}F-FDG PET/CT were independent and significant prognostic factors. Univariate and multivariate analyses revealed that the significant independent predictors of poor survival outcomes were the nonepithelioid histologic type, increased serum LDH, an NLR of ≥5.0, and a TLG of ≥525 g.[111]

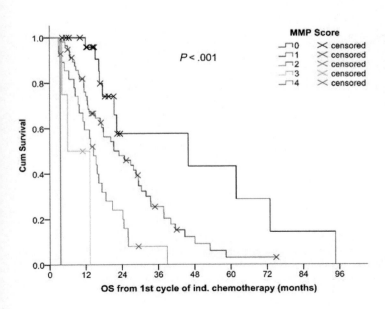

Fig. 3. MMP Score. Kaplan-Meier curve comparing overall survival (OS) according to the multimodality prognostic score (MMPS score) in patients treated with induction chemotherapy followed by MCR. Source: Opitz et al. 2015 unpublished data.

The problem with most of the scores so far is the lack of validation in independent cohorts and the inclusion of clinical variables being available before surgery to help decision-making for or against surgical resection.[112] For this purpose, the authors defined in 2012 a multimodality prognostic score (MMPS) to screen patients and define subgroups eligible or especially not eligible for surgery.[113] The items in the score consisted of tumor volume before chemotherapy (>500 mL), nonepithelioid histologic subtype, CRP greater than 30 mg/L before chemotherapy, and progressive disease after chemotherapy assessed by mRECIST criteria. The cutoff within this score was at 2 and the specificity of scores 3 and 4 was 100%. The median OS for patients with a score of 0, 1, and 2 was 34, 17, and 12 months, respectively, whereas patients with a score of 3 or 4 had a median OS of 4 months (**Fig. 3**). The knowledge gained from the MMPS is important for counseling

patients because it allows one to reliably identify patients who may have a good chance to benefit from multimodality therapy including surgery and to rule out those in whom aggressive treatment may even cause harm. With a score of 3 or higher, patients are not considered to profit from an MCR in a multimodality therapy approach.[113] This score was further validated in an independent cohort from Vienna (**Fig. 4**) treated with the identical multimodality concept,[113] so that currently the authors are prospectively evaluating the score as an inclusion criterion for clinical trials.[112] The comparison of MMPS score with EORTC score using ROC curve analysis at 2 years showed that the MMPS demonstrated a better predictive power for OS than the EORTC score.[10,113]

The recommendations from current BTS guidelines for the investigation and management of MPM[42] include the following (all grade D). Consider calculating a prognostic score in patients

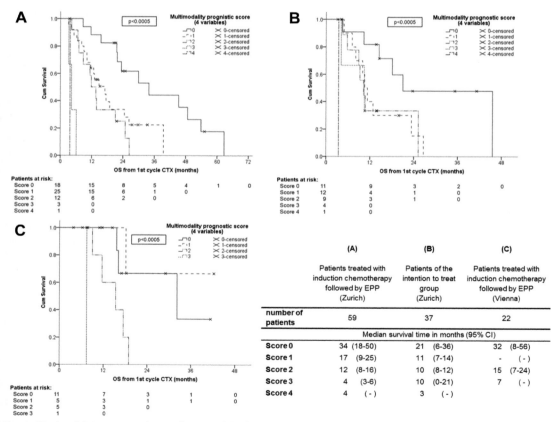

Fig. 4. Kaplan-Meier curve of overall survival (OS) in months of the multimodality prognostic score. (A) Patients treated with induction chemotherapy followed by extrapleural pneumonectomy (EPP; Zurich). (B) Patients of the intention-to-treat group (Zurich). (C) Patients treated with induction chemotherapy followed by EPP (Vienna). (*From* Opitz I, Friess M, Kestenholz P, et al. A new prognostic score supporting treatment allocation for multimodality therapy for malignant pleural mesothelioma: a review of 12 years' experience. J Thorac Oncol. 2015;10(11):1640; with permission.)

with MPM at diagnosis. Prognostic scores can provide useful survival information for patients and doctors but should not be used in treatment decision-making. When calculating a prognostic score, use one of the following: (a) the EORTC PS; (b) the CALGB score; (c) the mGPS; (d) the LENT score if a pleural effusion is present; (e) the decision tree analysis. The decision tree analysis scoring system is likely to be the most useful in routine clinical practice.[42] Future investigations needs to extend staging supplemental variables with validation of already available clinical prognostic indices (EORTC and CALGB scores) in combination with laboratory parameters or biomarkers to define the best surgical candidates, as recommended in the ASCO guidelines.[6]

SUMMARY

Currently there are no generally accepted criteria for patient selection for surgery within a multimodality treatment protocol, but patient selection remains the key parameter for surgical success and low morbidity and mortality. Among clinical, pathologic, and molecular prognostic factors studied in the past, the combination of several factors seems to be the most appropriate tool for decision-making, including also institutional experience and availability of therapy as well as factors such as the patient's choice of treatment. Preoperative identification of benefit from surgery comprising a summary of interdisciplinary preoperative workup includes many aspects in this decision-making process, including exact diagnosis, staging, validated prognostic scores, multimodal therapy options based on recommendations of the multidisciplinary tumor board, and prospective evaluation of these treatment allocation protocols, when selecting the appropriate therapy for patients in the future. In appropriately selected patients with an acceptable risk profile, surgical resection (extended P/D, P/D, or EPP) as part of a multimodality concept should still be offered if performed in high-volume and low-mortality centers, and in any case inclusion in clinical trials or large national or international registries is recommended.

Clinics Care Points

- Preoperative identification of benefit from surgery is contributed by clinical prognosticators (including age, gender, ECOG PS status, radiologic and surgical staging at baseline and after induction treatment, genetic and molecular factors, laboratory parameters) which, combined with consideration of QoL, are applied often in prognostic scores and

allow identification of selected patients for curative approach.
- Future prospective randomized trials must validate all of these approaches to select the best surgical candidates according to approved international guidelines.

DISCLOSURE

The authors have nothing to disclose.

REFERENCES

1. Stayner L, Welch LS, Lemen R. The worldwide pandemic of asbestos-related diseases. Annu Rev Public Health 2013;34:205–16.
2. Craighead JE. Epidemiology of mesothelioma and historical background. Recent Results Cancer Res 2011;189:13–25.
3. The Lancet Respiratory M. Pleural mesothelioma: tackling a deadly cancer. Lancet Respir Med 2019;7(2):99.
4. Bray F, Ferlay J, Soerjomataram I, et al. Global cancer statistics 2018: GLOBOCAN estimates of incidence and mortality worldwide for 36 cancers in 185 countries. CA Cancer J Clin 2018;68(6):394–424.
5. Bibby AC, Maskell NA. Current treatments and trials in malignant pleural mesothelioma. Clin Respir J 2018;12(7):2161–9.
6. Kindler HL, Ismaila N, Armato SG 3rd, et al. Treatment of malignant pleural mesothelioma: American Society of Clinical Oncology clinical practice guideline. J Clin Oncol 2018;36(13):1343–73.
7. Butchart EG, Ashcroft T, Barnsley WC, et al. Pleuropneumonectomy in the management of diffuse malignant mesothelioma of the pleura. Experience with 29 patients. Thorax 1976;31(1):15–24.
8. Scherpereel A, Astoul P, Baas P, et al. Guidelines of the European Respiratory Society and the European Society of Thoracic Surgeons for the management of malignant pleural mesothelioma. Eur Respir J 2010;35(3):479–95.
9. Edwards JG, Martin-Ucar AE, Stewart DJ, et al. Right extrapleural pneumonectomy for malignant mesothelioma via median sternotomy or thoracotomy? Short- and long-term results. Eur J Cardiothorac Surg 2007;31(5):759–64.
10. Curran D, Sahmoud T, Therasse P, et al. Prognostic factors in patients with pleural mesothelioma: the European Organization for Research and Treatment of Cancer experience. J Clin Oncol 1998;16(1):145–52.
11. Herndon JE, Green MR, Chahinian AP, et al. Factors predictive of survival among 337 patients with mesothelioma treated between 1984 and

1994 by the Cancer and Leukemia Group B. Chest 1998;113(3):723–31.

12. Edwards JG, Abrams KR, Leverment JN, et al. Prognostic factors for malignant mesothelioma in 142 patients: validation of CALGB and EORTC prognostic scoring systems. Thorax 2000;55(9): 731–5.

13. Gonlugur U, Gonlugur TE. Prognostic factors for 100 patients with malignant pleural mesothelioma. Arch Environ Occup Health 2010;65(2):65–9.

14. Gillezeau CN, van Gerwen M, Ramos J, et al. Biomarkers for malignant pleural mesothelioma: a meta-analysis. Carcinogenesis 2019;40(11): 1320–31.

15. Pinato DJ, Mauri FA, Ramakrishnan R, et al. Inflammation-based prognostic indices in malignant pleural mesothelioma. J Thorac Oncol 2012;7(3):587–94.

16. Ghanim B, Hoda MA, Winter MP, et al. Pretreatment serum C-reactive protein levels predict benefit from multimodality treatment including radical surgery in malignant pleural mesothelioma: a retrospective multicenter analysis. Ann Surg 2012;256(2): 357–62.

17. Ghanim B, Hoda MA, Klikovits T, et al. Circulating fibrinogen is a prognostic and predictive biomarker in malignant pleural mesothelioma. Br J Cancer 2014;110(4):984–90.

18. Fleisher LA, Beckman JA, Brown KA, et al. ACC/ AHA 2007 guidelines on perioperative cardiovascular evaluation and care for noncardiac surgery: a report of the American College of Cardiology/ American Heart Association Task Force on Practice Guidelines (Writing Committee to Revise the 2002 Guidelines on Perioperative Cardiovascular Evaluation for Noncardiac Surgery) developed in collaboration with the American Society of Echocardiography, American Society of Nuclear Cardiology, Heart Rhythm Society, Society of Cardiovascular Anesthesiologists, Society for Cardiovascular Angiography and Interventions, Society for Vascular Medicine and Biology, and Society for Vascular Surgery. J Am Coll Cardiol 2007; 50(17):e159–241.

19. Culver BH, Graham BL, Coates AL, et al. Recommendations for a standardized pulmonary function report. An official American Thoracic Society technical statement. Am J Respir Crit Care Med 2017; 196(11):1463–72.

20. Flores RM, Riedel E, Donington JS, et al. Frequency of use and predictors of cancer-directed surgery in the management of malignant pleural mesothelioma in a community-based (Surveillance, Epidemiology, and End Results [SEER]) population. J Thorac Oncol 2010;5(10): 1649–54.

21. Taioli E, Wolf AS, Camacho-Rivera M, et al. Determinants of survival in malignant pleural mesothelioma: a surveillance, epidemiology, and end results (SEER) study of 14,228 patients. PLoS One 2015;10(12):e0145039.

22. Ettinger DS, Akerley W, Borghaei H, et al. Malignant pleural mesothelioma. J Natl Compr Cancer Netw 2012;10(1):26–41.

23. Yang CJ, Yan BW, Meyerhoff RR, et al. Impact of age on long-term outcomes of surgery for malignant pleural mesothelioma. Clin Lung Cancer 2016;17(5):419–26.

24. Meyerhoff RR, Yang CF, Speicher PJ, et al. Impact of mesothelioma histologic subtype on outcomes in the Surveillance, Epidemiology, and End Results database. J Surg Res 2015;196(1):23–32.

25. Amin W, Linkov F, Landsittel D, et al. Factors influencing malignant mesothelioma survival: a retrospective review of the National Mesothelioma Virtual Bank cohort [version 2; peer review: 2 approved, 1 approved with reservations]. F1000Res 2018;7:1184.

26. Bovolato P, Casadio C, Bille A, et al. Does surgery improve survival of patients with malignant pleural mesothelioma?: a multicenter retrospective analysis of 1365 consecutive patients. J Thorac Oncol 2014;9(3):390–6.

27. Zhuo M, Zheng Q, Chi Y, et al. Survival analysis via nomogram of surgical patients with malignant pleural mesothelioma in the Surveillance, Epidemiology, and End Results database. Thorac Cancer 2019;10(5):1193–202.

28. Taioli E, Wolf AS, Camacho-Rivera M, et al. Women with malignant pleural mesothelioma have a threefold better survival rate than men. Ann Thorac Surg 2014;98(3):1020–4.

29. Linton A, Pavlakis N, O'Connell R, et al. Factors associated with survival in a large series of patients with malignant pleural mesothelioma in New South Wales. Br J Cancer 2014;111(9):1860–9.

30. Pinton G, Brunelli E, Murer B, et al. Estrogen receptor-beta affects the prognosis of human malignant mesothelioma. Cancer Res 2009;69(11): 4598–604.

31. Van Gerwen M, Alpert N, Wolf A, et al. Prognostic factors of survival in patients with malignant pleural mesothelioma: an analysis of the National Cancer Database. Carcinogenesis 2019;40(4): 529–36.

32. van Meerbeeck JP, Gaafar R, Manegold C, et al. Randomized Phase III Study of Cisplatin With or Without Raltitrexed in Patients With Malignant Pleural Mesothelioma: An Intergroup Study of the European Organisation for Research and Treatment of Cancer Lung Cancer Group and the National Cancer Institute of Canada. J Clin Oncol 2005;23(28):6881–9.

33. Ceresoli GL, Grosso F, Zucali PA, et al. Prognostic factors in elderly patients with malignant pleural

mesothelioma: results of a multicenter survey. Br J Cancer 2014;111(2):220–6.

34. Chen N, Liu S, Huang L, et al. Prognostic significance of neutrophil-to-lymphocyte ratio in patients with malignant pleural mesothelioma: a meta-analysis. Oncotarget 2017;8(34):57460–9.

35. Bibby AC, Dorn P, Psallidas I, et al. ERS/EACTS statement on the management of malignant pleural effusions. Eur Respir J 2018;52(1):1800349.

36. Ghanim B, Rosenmayr A, Stockhammer P, et al. Tumour cell PD-L1 expression is prognostic in patients with malignant pleural effusion: the impact of C-reactive protein and immune-checkpoint inhibition. Sci Rep 2020;10(1):5784.

37. Chen ZJ, Gaudino G, Pass HI, et al. Diagnostic and prognostic biomarkers for malignant mesothelioma: an update. Transl Lung Cancer Res 2017;6(3):259–69.

38. Sun HH, Vaynblat A, Pass HI. Diagnosis and prognosis—review of biomarkers for mesothelioma. Ann Transl Med 2017;5(11):244.

39. Wu T, Zhang W, Yang G, et al. HMGB1 overexpression as a prognostic factor for survival in cancer: a meta-analysis and systematic review. Oncotarget 2016;7(31):50417–27.

40. Tabata C, Shibata E, Tabata R, et al. Serum HMGB1 as a prognostic marker for malignant pleural mesothelioma. BMC Cancer 2013;13:205.

41. Yamagishi T, Fujimoto N, Nishi H, et al. Prognostic significance of the lymphocyte-to-monocyte ratio in patients with malignant pleural mesothelioma. Lung Cancer 2015;90(1):111–7.

42. Woolhouse I, Bishop L, Darlison L, et al. British Thoracic Society Guideline for the investigation and management of malignant pleural mesothelioma. Thorax 2018;73(Suppl 1):i1–30.

43. Frauenfelder T, Kestenholz P, Hunziker R, et al. Use of computed tomography and positron emission tomography/computed tomography for staging of local extent in patients with malignant pleural mesothelioma. J Comput Assist Tomogr 2015;39(2):160–5.

44. Martini K, Meier A, Opitz I, et al. Diagnostic accuracy of sequential co-registered PET+MR in comparison to PET/CT in local thoracic staging of malignant pleural mesothelioma. Lung Cancer 2016;94:40–5.

45. Wang ZJ, Reddy GP, Gotway MB, et al. Malignant pleural mesothelioma: evaluation with CT, MR imaging, and PET. Radiographics 2004;24(1):105–19.

46. Rusch VW, Venkatraman ES. Important prognostic factors in patients with malignant pleural mesothelioma, managed surgically. Ann Thorac Surg 1999;68(5):1799–804.

47. Frauenfelder T, Tutic M, Weder W, et al. Volumetry: an alternative to assess therapy response for malignant pleural mesothelioma? Eur Respir J 2011;38(1):162–8.

48. Armato SG 3rd, Blyth KG, Keating JJ, et al. Imaging in pleural mesothelioma: A review of the 13th international conference of the international mesothelioma interest group. Lung Cancer 2016;101:48–58.

49. Lee HY, Hyun SH, Lee KS, et al. Volume-based parameter of 18)F-FDG PET/CT in malignant pleural mesothelioma: prediction of therapeutic response and prognostic implications. Ann Surg Oncol 2010;17(10):2787–94.

50. Rusch VW, Chansky K, Kindler HL, et al. The IASLC Mesothelioma Staging Project: proposals for the M descriptors and for revision of the TNM stage groupings in the forthcoming (eighth) edition of the TNM Classification for Mesothelioma. J Thorac Oncol 2016;11(12):2112–9.

51. Nowak AK, Chansky K, Rice DC, et al. The IASLC mesothelioma staging project: proposals for revisions of the T descriptors in the forthcoming eighth edition of the TNM classification for pleural mesothelioma. J Thorac Oncol 2016;11(12):2089–99.

52. Sugarbaker DJ, Flores RM, Jaklitsch MT, et al. Resection margins, extrapleural nodal status, and cell type determine postoperative long-term survival in trimodality therapy of malignant pleural mesothelioma: results in 183 patients. J Thorac Cardiovasc Surg 1999;117(1):54–63 [discussion: 63–65].

53. Sugarbaker DJ, Strauss GM, Lynch TJ, et al. Node status has prognostic significance in the multimodality therapy of diffuse, malignant mesothelioma. J Clin Oncol 1993;11(6):1172–8.

54. Scherpereel A, Astoul P, Baas P, et al. [Guidelines of the European Respiratory Society and the European Society of Thoracic Surgeons for the management of malignant pleural mesothelioma]. Zhongguo Fei Ai Za Zhi 2010;13(10):C23–45.

55. Rice D, Chansky K, Nowak A, et al. The IASLC mesothelioma staging project: proposals for revisions of the N descriptors in the forthcoming eighth edition of the TNM classification for pleural mesothelioma. J Thorac Oncol 2016;11(12):2100–11.

56. Verma V, Wegner RE, Stahl JM, et al. Impact of detecting occult pathologic nodal disease during resection for malignant pleural mesothelioma. Clin Lung Cancer 2020;21(4):e274–85.

57. Sinha S, Swift AJ, Kamil MA, et al. The role of imaging in malignant pleural mesothelioma: an update after the 2018 BTS guidelines. Clin Radiol 2020;75(6):423–32.

58. van Klaveren RJ, Aerts JG, de Bruin H, et al. Inadequacy of the RECIST criteria for response evaluation in patients with malignant pleural mesothelioma. Lung Cancer 2004;43(1):63–9.

59. Byrne MJ, Nowak AK. Modified RECIST criteria for assessment of response in malignant pleural mesothelioma. Ann Oncol 2004;15(2):257–60.

60. Bonomi M, De Filippis C, Lopci E, et al. Clinical staging of malignant pleural mesothelioma: current perspectives. Lung Cancer 2017;8:127–39.

61. Armato SG 3rd, Oxnard GR, MacMahon H, et al. Measurement of mesothelioma on thoracic CT scans: a comparison of manual and computer-assisted techniques. Med Phys 2004;31(5):1105–15.

62. Kindler HL, Ismaila N, Hassan R. Treatment of malignant pleural mesothelioma: American Society of Clinical Oncology clinical practice guideline summary. J Oncol Pract 2018;14(4):256–64.

63. Krug LM, Pass HI, Rusch VW, et al. Multicenter phase II trial of neoadjuvant pemetrexed plus cisplatin followed by extrapleural pneumonectomy and radiation for malignant pleural mesothelioma. J Clin Oncol 2009;27(18):3007–13.

64. Gudmundsson E, Straus CM, Armato SG 3rd. Deep convolutional neural networks for the automated segmentation of malignant pleural mesothelioma on computed tomography scans. J Med Imaging (Bellingham) 2018;5(3):034503.

65. Rusch VW, Gill R, Mitchell A, et al. A multicenter study of volumetric computed tomography for staging malignant pleural mesothelioma. Ann Thorac Surg 2016;102(4):1059–66.

66. Liu F, Zhao B, Krug LM, et al. Assessment of therapy responses and prediction of survival in malignant pleural mesothelioma through computer-aided volumetric measurement on computed tomography scans. J Thorac Oncol 2010;5(6):879–84.

67. Plathow C, Klopp M, Thieke C, et al. Therapy response in malignant pleural mesothelioma-role of MRI using RECIST, modified RECIST and volumetric approaches in comparison with CT. Eur Radiol 2008;18(8):1635–43.

68. Labby ZE, Nowak AK, Dignam JJ, et al. Disease volumes as a marker for patient response in malignant pleural mesothelioma. Ann Oncol 2013;24(4):999–1005.

69. Armato SG 3rd, Francis RJ, Katz SI, et al. Imaging in pleural mesothelioma: A review of the 14th International Conference of the International Mesothelioma Interest Group. Lung Cancer 2019;130:108–14.

70. Labby ZE, Armato SG 3rd, Dignam JJ, et al. Lung volume measurements as a surrogate marker for patient response in malignant pleural mesothelioma. J Thorac Oncol 2013;8(4):478–86.

71. Pass HI, Temeck BK, Kranda K, et al. Preoperative tumor volume is associated with outcome in malignant pleural mesothelioma. J Thorac Cardiovasc Surg 1998;115(2):310–7 [discussion: 317–318].

72. Sensakovic WF, Armato SG 3rd, Straus C, et al. Computerized segmentation and measurement of malignant pleural mesothelioma. Med Phys 2011;38(1):238–44.

73. Gill RR, Richards WG, Yeap BY, et al. Epithelial malignant pleural mesothelioma after extrapleural pneumonectomy: stratification of survival with CT-derived tumor volume. AJR Am J Roentgenol 2012;198(2):359–63.

74. Pavic M, Bogowicz M, Wurms X, et al. Influence of inter-observer delineation variability on radiomics stability in different tumor sites. Acta Oncol 2018;57(8):1070–4.

75. Weber MA, Bock M, Plathow C, et al. Asbestos-related pleural disease: value of dedicated magnetic resonance imaging techniques. Invest Radiol 2004;39(9):554–64.

76. Burt BM, Lee HS, Raghuram AC, et al. Preoperative prediction of unresectability in malignant pleural mesothelioma. J Thorac Cardiovasc Surg 2019;159(6):2512–20.e1.

77. Armato SG 3rd, Labby ZE, Coolen J, et al. Imaging in pleural mesothelioma: a review of the 11th International Conference of the International Mesothelioma Interest Group. Lung Cancer 2013;82(2):190–6.

78. Lim JH, Choi JY, Im Y, et al. Prognostic value of SUVmax on 18F-fluorodeoxyglucose PET/CT scan in patients with malignant pleural mesothelioma. PLoS One 2020;15(2):e0229299.

79. Schwartz RM, Lieberman-Cribbin W, Wolf A, et al. Systematic review of quality of life following pleurectomy decortication and extrapleural pneumonectomy for malignant pleural mesothelioma. BMC cancer 2018;18(1):1188.

80. Rena O, Casadio C. Extrapleural pneumonectomy for early stage malignant pleural mesothelioma: a harmful procedure. Lung Cancer 2012;77(1):151–5.

81. Ploenes T, Osei-Agyemang T, Krohn A, et al. Changes in lung function after surgery for mesothelioma. Asian Cardiovasc Thorac Ann 2013;21(1):48–55.

82. Nakas A, Waller D. Predictors of long-term survival following radical surgery for malignant pleural mesothelioma. Eur J Cardiothorac Surg 2014;46(3):380–5 [discussion: 385].

83. Galateau-Salle F, Churg A, Roggli V, et al. The 2015 World Health Organization classification of tumors of the pleura: advances since the 2004 classification. J Thorac Oncol 2016;11(2):142–54.

84. Woodard GA, Jablons DM. Surgery for pleural mesothelioma, when it is indicated and why: arguments against surgery for malignant pleural mesothelioma. Transl Lung Cancer Res 2020;9(Suppl 1):S86–91.

85. Travis WD, Brambilla E, Burke AP, et al. Introduction to The 2015 World Health Organization classification of tumors of the lung, pleura, thymus, and heart. J Thorac Oncol 2015;10(9):1240–2.

86. Bilecz A, Stockhammer P, Theegarten D, et al. Comparative analysis of prognostic histopathologic parameters in subtypes of epithelioid pleural mesothelioma. Histopathology 2020;77(1):55–66.

87. Musk AW, Olsen N, Alfonso H, et al. Predicting survival in malignant mesothelioma. Eur Respir J 2011; 38(6):1420–4.

88. Saddoughi SA, Abdelsattar ZM, Blackmon SH. National trends in the epidemiology of malignant pleural mesothelioma: a national cancer data base study. Ann Thorac Surg 2018;105(2):432–7.

89. Nakas A, Trousse DS, Martin-Ucar AE, et al. Open lung-sparing surgery for malignant pleural mesothelioma: the benefits of a radical approach within multimodality therapy. Eur J Cardiothorac Surg 2008;34(4):886–91.

90. Neragi-Miandoab S, Richards WG, Sugarbaker DJ. Morbidity, mortality, mean survival, and the impact of histology on survival after pleurectomy in 64 patients with malignant pleural mesothelioma. Int J Surg 2008;6(4):293–7.

91. Jean D, Daubriac J, Le Pimpec-Barthes F, et al. Molecular changes in mesothelioma with an impact on prognosis and treatment. Arch Pathol Lab Med 2012;136(3):277–93.

92. Baumann F, Flores E, Napolitano A, et al. Mesothelioma patients with germline BAP1 mutations have 7-fold improved long-term survival. Carcinogenesis 2015;36(1):76–81.

93. McGregor SM, Dunning R, Hyjek E, et al. BAP1 facilitates diagnostic objectivity, classification, and prognostication in malignant pleural mesothelioma. Hum Pathol 2015;46(11):1670–8.

94. Bartel DP. MicroRNAs: Genomics, biogenesis, mechanism, and function. Cell 2004;116(2):281–97.

95. Ambros V. The functions of animal microRNAs. Nature 2004;431(7006):350–5.

96. Kirschner MB, Cheng YY, Armstrong NJ, et al. MiRscore: a novel 6-microRNA signature that predicts survival outcomes in patients with malignant pleural mesothelioma. Mol Oncol 2015;9(3):715–26.

97. Opitz I, Soltermann A, Abaecherli M, et al. PTEN expression is a strong predictor of survival in mesothelioma patients. Eur J Cardiothorac Surg 2008; 33(3):502–6.

98. Bitanihirwe BK, Meerang M, Friess M, et al. PI3K/mTOR signaling in mesothelioma patients treated with induction chemotherapy followed by extrapleural pneumonectomy. J Thorac Oncol 2014;9(2):239–47.

99. Schramm A, Opitz I, Thies S, et al. Prognostic significance of epithelial-mesenchymal transition in malignant pleural mesothelioma. Eur J Cardiothorac Surg 2010;37(3):566–72.

100. Kuroda A, Matsumoto S, Fukuda A, et al. The mTOR signaling pathway is associated with the prognosis of malignant pleural mesothelioma after multimodality therapy. Anticancer Res 2019; 39(11):6241–7.

101. Otterstrom C, Soltermann A, Opitz I, et al. CD74: a new prognostic factor for patients with malignant pleural mesothelioma. Br J Cancer 2014;110(8):2040–6.

102. Thies S, Friess M, Frischknecht L, et al. Expression of the stem cell factor nestin in malignant pleural mesothelioma is associated with poor prognosis. PLoS One 2015;10(9):e0139312.

103. Meerang M, Berard K, Friess M, et al. Low Merlin expression and high Survivin labeling index are indicators for poor prognosis in patients with malignant pleural mesothelioma. Mol Oncol 2016;10(8): 1255–65.

104. Nguyen BH, Montgomery R, Fadia M, et al. PD-L1 expression associated with worse survival outcome in malignant pleural mesothelioma. Asia Pac J Clin Oncol 2018;14(1):69–73.

105. Sandri A, Guerrera F, Roffinella M, et al. Validation of EORTC and CALGB prognostic models in surgical patients submitted to diagnostic, palliative or curative surgery for malignant pleural mesothelioma. J Thorac Dis 2016;8(8):2121–7.

106. Leuzzi G, Rea F, Spaggiari L, et al. Prognostic score of long-term survival after surgery for malignant pleural mesothelioma: a multicenter analysis. Ann Thorac Surg 2015;100(3):890–7.

107. Rusch VW, Giroux D, Kennedy C, et al. Initial analysis of the international association for the study of lung cancer mesothelioma database. J Thorac Oncol 2012;7(11):1631–9.

108. Pass HI, Giroux D, Kennedy C, et al. Supplementary prognostic variables for pleural mesothelioma: a report from the IASLC staging committee. J Thorac Oncol 2014;9(6):856–64.

109. Clive AO, Kahan BC, Hooper CE, et al. Predicting survival in malignant pleural effusion: development and validation of the LENT prognostic score. Thorax 2014;69(12):1098–104.

110. Brims FJ, Meniawy TM, Duffus I, et al. A novel clinical prediction model for prognosis in malignant pleural mesothelioma using decision tree analysis. J Thorac Oncol 2016;11(4):573–82.

111. Doi H, Kuribayashi K, Kitajima K, et al. Development of a novel prognostic risk classification system for malignant pleural mesothelioma. Clin Lung Cancer 2020;21(1):66–74.e2.

112. Opitz I, Weder W. Pleural mesothelioma: is the surgeon still there? Ann Oncol 2018;29(8):1710–7.

113. Opitz I, Friess M, Kestenholz P, et al. A new prognostic score supporting treatment allocation for multimodality therapy for malignant pleural mesothelioma: a review of 12 years' experience. J Thorac Oncol 2015;10(11):1634–41.

Extended Pleurectomy and Decortication for Malignant Pleural Mesothelioma

R. Taylor Ripley, MD

KEYWORDS

• Mesothelioma • Pleurectomy • Decortication • Lung-sparing • Asbestos

KEY POINTS

- Extended pleurectomy and decortication (ePD) is a lung-sparing surgery that indicates a visceral and parietal pleurectomy with the resection of the diaphragm and/or pericardium.
- The goal of curative surgical resection is to achieve a macroscopic complete resection, which may be accomplished by ePD.
- The goal of the visceral decortication is to remove all tumor, to expand the trapped lung, and to minimize air leaks.
- Despite lack of direct comparisons, ePD has a lower perioperative mortality, similar long-term survival, and better tolerance in patients with lower performance status versus extrapleural pneumonectomy.

INTRODUCTION

Malignant mesothelioma arises from the pleura, peritoneum, pericardium, or tunica vaginalis. Malignant pleural mesothelioma (MPM) is the most common type of malignant mesothelioma, which occurs in 3000 patients per year in the United States. Although other causes exist, asbestos exposure is the most common cause. Although MPM is often a rapidly fatal malignancy, multimodality therapy with surgery and chemotherapy may result in long-term survival in selected patients. Surgery is a component of the diagnosis, staging, and treatment of MPM.[1] The National Comprehensive Cancer Network, the European Society for Medical Oncology, and American Society of Clinical Oncology have published recent guidelines that recommend surgery as part of the diagnosis and treatment of MPM for curative and palliative intents.[2–4]

The goal of curative surgical resection is to achieve a macroscopic complete resection.[5] Because MPM covers all surfaces in the chest, negative margins are not feasible; therefore, achieving an R0 resection is not the goal of the curative surgery. Recently, the National Cancer Institute (NCI), the International Association for the Study of Lung Cancer (IASLC), and the Mesothelioma Applied Research Foundation (MARF) proposed standardizing the surgical procedures for MPM. Surgery is performed with either a lung-sparing surgery called an extended pleurectomy/decortication (ePD) or a lung-sacrificing surgery called an extrapleural pneumonectomy (EPP).[6] A pleurectomy and decortication indicates a visceral and parietal pleurectomy, whereas the extended descriptor includes the resection of the diaphragm and/or pericardium. Despite standardization of these definitions, whether partial diaphragm or pericardial resections qualify as extended is debatable. Regardless of the nuances

Department of Surgery, Division of General Thoracic Surgery, The Michael E. DeBakey Department of Surgery, Baylor College of Medicine, Houston, TX 77030, USA
E-mail address: R.Taylor.Ripley@bcm.edu

Thorac Surg Clin 30 (2020) 451–460
https://doi.org/10.1016/j.thorsurg.2020.07.002
1547-4127/20/© 2020 Elsevier Inc. All rights reserved.

of the definitions and the differences in the operations, the goal of an ePD is to render the patient with no evidence of visible, palpable, or viable tumor without resection of the lung.

This article describes the ePD. This operation is almost always part of multimodality therapy that includes chemotherapy and possibly radiotherapy. These topics are covered in other articles in this issue so they are not discussed here. However, ePD is a component of a treatment strategy that includes a multidisciplinary team.

ANATOMY

MPM involves the entire pleura and encases the lung as it progresses. MPM initially forms small, independent nodules that convalesce into sheets of tumor. The pleural space is obliterated and filled with tumor and effusions. The tumor invades adjacent structures such as the chest wall, diaphragm, and pericardium. MPM spreads to lymph nodes in the lungs, mediastinum, and chest wall. Although less common, MPM does metastasize to distant organs. The extent of the disease is defined based on stage. The staging of MPM is described in a separate article in this issue.

CLINICAL PRESENTATION

Shortness of breath, fatigue, and chest wall pain are common presenting symptoms. Patients are often symptomatic for months before diagnosis. Prior thoracentesis with cytology may have been performed; however, the cytologic diagnostic accuracy for MPM from pleural fluid is low and the disease may not be suspected, so the effusions usually recur.[7,8] Chest wall pain is an ominous symptom that is associated with chest wall invasion. Chest retraction and excessive weight loss are signs of advanced disease.

DIAGNOSIS AND PREOPERATIVE EVALUATION

For newly diagnosed MPM, confirmation of the diagnosis and subtype, establishment of the extent or clinic stage, and assessment the physiologic status of the patient are performed. This extensive evaluation is necessary to develop the most appropriate treatment plan.

Recurrent effusions are often managed with diagnostic biopsies by video-assisted thoracoscopic surgery (VATS). Confirmation of the disorder or rebiopsy is required to establish the diagnosis with histologic subtype when patients are referred to centers specializing in MPM. Given the implications of the diagnosis and treatment, repeated VATS biopsies are justifiable before

treatment recommendations. After diagnosis, the next goal is to establish the stage and extent of disease.[9] PET scans, computed tomography (CT) scans, and MRI assist in determining resectability. The PET scan evaluates mediastinal lymph nodes and distant sites.[10] The MRI assists with identifying chest wall, diaphragm, aortic, and mediastinal invasion. However, neither CT nor MRI is superior for detection of chest wall invasion; therefore, MRI can be omitted.

Extended staging with invasive biopsies and confirmation of the disease are important to identify subsets of patients with advanced disease that is not apparent based on imaging.[11] Diagnostic laparoscopy reveals disease in up to 18% of patients even without 18F-fluorodeoxyglucose avidity in the peritoneum. Mediastinoscopy helps identify some patients with nodal disease; however, the pattern of nodal spread does not mirror lung cancer, so most nodal disease is not identified on mediastinoscopy. It is useful for excluding marginal operative candidates who have suspicious disease in stations 2, 4, or 7. Mediastinoscopy, diagnostic laparoscopy, and repeat VATS biopsy can be performed in 1 operative setting.

Assessment of cardiopulmonary reserve is critical for minimizing perioperative risk. Pulmonary assessment includes pulmonary function tests (PFTs) and ventilation perfusion (VQ) nuclear scans. Measurement of diffusion of limited carbon monoxide (DLco) is necessary because prior asbestos exposure may result in asbestosis with restricted pulmonary diffusion. The patients often have severe reduction in pulmonary function; however, if the perfusion to the affected side is low, they can tolerate removal of the lung or they may improve with decortication of the disease. Cardiovascular evaluation consists of at least an echocardiogram, but, for patients with comorbidities, a formal cardiology consultation is recommended. Once all components of this evaluation have been completed, treatment recommendations may include surgery, chemotherapy, radiotherapy, multimodality therapy, or palliative care.[4]

OPERATIVE APPROACH
Preoperative Planning and Patient Positioning

An epidural catheter is placed in all patients. An arterial line is placed. A central venous catheter is used selectively. A pulmonary artery (PA) catheter is generally not used because of the risk of transection if the operation is converted to an EPP.

Patients are intubated with a double-lumen endotracheal tube. A flexible bronchoscopy is unnecessary given that endobronchial disease is rare in MPM. The patient remains on 2-lung ventilation as long as possible to decrease the risk of barotrauma to the contralateral lung. Once the operation is completed, the double-lumen tube is changed to a single-lumen tube and a therapeutic flexible bronchoscopy is performed to clear all secretions.

The patient is placed in standard lateral decubitus position with slight anterior rotation of the hip to facilitate exposure to the diaphragm (**Fig. 1**).

Step 1: Incision and Muscle Preservation

An extended posterolateral S-shaped thoracotomy is marked with incorporation of prior VATS port sites if feasible. If these sites are distant to the incision, they are marked and resected independently. If tumor is not palpable in the port sites, frozen section analysis is performed on the excised skin. If tumor is present, all soft tissue under these incisions is excised into the chest cavity.

The central portion of the incision is opened. The latissimus dorsi is mobilized from the subcutaneous tissue and chest wall to provide access to the sixth rib. The serratus anterior is lifted off the sixth rib. The muscles are retracted with a Balfour retractor. Postoperatively, the spaces outside the chest wall can communicate with the pleural space, which may result in a seroma. To prevent this complication, the dissection is limited to only

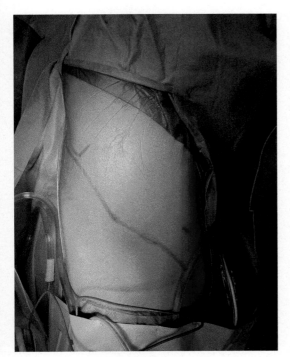

Fig. 1. Right extended posterolateral thoracotomy with incorporation of prior VATS port site incisions.

the sixth rib, the intercostal muscles are preserved during resection of the rib, the intercostal muscles are sutured together when closing the chest, and the latissimus dorsi and the serratus anterior are parachuted onto the intercostal muscles to create a watertight seal. These muscles do not require transection for adequate exposure. Preservation allows management of residual thoracic cavity space if complications occur.

Step 2: Development of the Extrapleural Plane

After exposure of the sixth rib, the periosteum is scored and the rib is resected in the subperiosteal space. The intercostal muscle is lifted with an Allis retractor and the plane underneath the muscle is developed (**Fig. 2**). With the surgeon's fingertips upward, this plane is extended in all directions to start the parietal pleurectomy. If this dissection is not possible, chest wall invasion may be present and the tumor is potentially unresectable. Alternatively, if the pleura is removed from the chest wall easily, the incision is extended. Additional counterincisions of the chest wall are not necessary.

Step 3: Mobilization of the Posterior and Apical Parietal Pleura

The poster, apical, and anterior pleural dissections are usually easier than the inferior pleura and diaphragm. These dissections are performed by developing these planes to the pulmonary hilum from each direction.

The posterior pleural dissection on the right is developed from the chest wall, to the azygous, over the esophagus, to the posterior hilum. On the left, the dissection proceeds over the descending thoracic aorta. Careful attention is required to avoid inadvertently dissecting under the aorta and disrupting the segmental branches. If the anterior plane of the aorta is difficult to identify, the tumor may be unresectable. However, developing this plane from the aortic arch and diaphragm and connecting these 2 areas can facilitate this dissection. The fibrous adhesions between the pleura and the hilum require sharp dissection to completely mobilize the parietal pleura to the visceral pleura. During this dissection, lymph nodes are resected from levels 7, 8, and 9.

The apical pleural dissection removes the disease from the chest wall superior to the incision, around the apex of the chest, and to the superior mediastinum. Dissection of the mediastinal pleura is performed by pushing the structures into the mediastinum rather than pulling the pleura of the mediastinum to avoid injury to vessels, the recurrent laryngeal nerves (RLNs), lymphatics, and

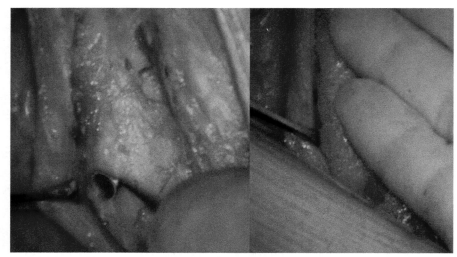

Fig. 2. The intercostal muscle is lifted to develop the plane underneath the muscle. This plane is extended in all directions with the surgeon's hand.

airways. Pushing these structures off the mediastinal pleura rather than pulling helps minimize traction injuries. On the right, this dissection is completed once the azygous is identified and mobilized off the superior hilum. Level 4R lymph node dissection is performed. On the left, the apical dissection crosses over the aortic arch onto the left main PA. Traction on the vagus or cautery near the arch can injure the RLN. During this dissection, levels 5 and 6 lymph node dissections are performed.

Step 4: Mobilization of the Anterior Parietal Pleura

The anterior pleural dissection removes the parietal pleura off the chest wall, from the thymus, to the pericardium (**Fig. 3**). The anterior chest wall dissection extends over the pericardial fat into the pericardiosternal recess. This fat is swept toward the lung until the parietal pleura of the pericardium is identified. Internal mammary, pericardial fat pad, and diaphragmatic nodes are removed during this step. Once the dissection reaches the pericardium, the pleura is peeled off the fibrous pericardium to the pulmonary veins. If the disease invades the pericardium, separation of the fibrous and serous pericardium may complete the dissection. If removal is not possible without complete pericardial resection, the anterior dissection is stopped and resected later in the operation to prevent retraction to the contralateral side and hemodynamic instability. The anterior dissection connects to the apical dissection between the superior pulmonary vein (SPV) and the main PA on the left. On the right, the SPV, the

junction of the superior vena cava, and the truncus branch of the PA connect the anterior and apical dissections. The phrenic nerve is transected at this location if involved with disease. If possible, the phrenic is spared; however, its function after a diaphragm pleurectomy, and certainly after resection, is questionable. Level 10 lymph nodes are removed from both sides at this time.

Once the posterior, apical, and anterior pleural dissections are performed, the hilum is circumferentially exposed in all directions other than inferior to the inferior pulmonary vein (IPV). Completing these dissections off the mainstem bronchus, the SPV and IPV, and the PA during this part of the operation sets up the completion of the visceral

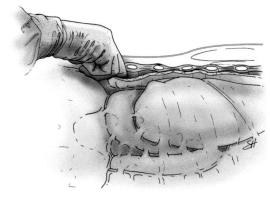

Fig. 3. The parietal pleurectomy is started with removal of the disease from the chest wall at the incision. This dissection is developed in all directions before extending the incision and placing the thoracic retractor. (© 2020 Baylor College of Medicine.)

pleurectomy. If the dissection does not completely expose the hilum, the visceral dissection approaches the pulmonary arteries and veins from more difficult directions.

Step 5: Mobilization of the Inferior Pleura and Resection of the Diaphragm

Resection of the inferior pleura includes the chest wall, the diaphragm, and mediastinal pleura between the IPV and the medial diaphragm. Performing this resection appropriately is critical to the reconstruction of the diaphragm. The inferior chest wall dissection includes the part of the posterior and apical dissections that connect to the costophrenic angle and the pericardium, respectively. This dissection begins with resection of all of the chest wall disease circumferentially to the diaphragmatic attachments.

The goal of the resection of the diaphragm is preservation of as much muscle as possible even though its function is questionable after this operation. The disease dictates the depth of resection. Beginning in the anterior sulcus is usually the easiest. If the pleura peels off the muscular diaphragm, most of the diaphragm other than the central tendon may be spared. If the muscle is partially invaded, then a partial-thickness resection of the muscle is performed (**Fig. 4**). If the disease invasion is extensive, the diaphragm is avulsed from the chest wall and completely resected. If the peritoneum is opened, it should be closed to prevent spread of tumor cells into the abdomen. Anteriorly, removal of the diaphragmatic disease exposes the angle between the diaphragm and pericardium. Posteriorly, the disease is peeled off above the esophagus on the right and above the aorta on the left. Often the muscle

can be preserved in 1 area, but not in others; therefore, significant variability in this step exists.

Eventually, peeling the disease off the muscle is no longer possible. At this point, resection of the diaphragm is easier from the abdominal side. The diaphragm is opened at the most lateral point and this opening is extended anteriorly and posteriorly to the mediastinum while preserving as much muscle as possible. On the right, avoiding injury to the spleen is critical. On the left, the right hepatic vein is encountered as the adhesions between the liver and diaphragm are removed. The peritoneum at the base of the diaphragm is scored about 1 to 2 cm lateral to the mediastinum. The diaphragm medial to this line provides a cuff to sew the patch to help prevent herniation (**Fig. 5**). Next, the thoracic portion of this diaphragm cuff is developed. The anterior and posterior pleural dissections are connected below the IPV by removing the inferior mediastinal pleura from the aorta and esophagus on the left and the azygous and esophagus on the right. The pleura is peeled off the medial diaphragm for 1 to 2 cm, which corresponds to the same line marked on the abdominal side of the diaphragm. Now, the medial diaphragm is transected with cautery while applying clips to the diaphragm edge to prevent bleeding (**Fig. 6**). Extreme care is required during this transection because tension on the phrenic veins can result in an avulsion injury that tears the inferior vena cava (IVC) into the abdomen (**Fig. 7**). This injury is possible from either side, and control of IVC bleeding is extremely difficult. At this point, the diaphragm resection is completed.

Often, developing the mediastinal pleura between the IPV and the diaphragm is not accessible by this method because the disease is too thick to expose this area (**Fig. 8**). An alternative approach is to start the visceral decortication on the base of the lung to approach the IPV (**Fig. 9**). This

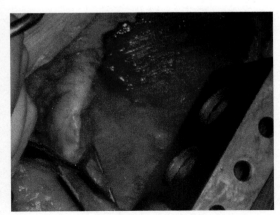

Fig. 4. When the disease is not invading the diaphragm, the muscular diaphragm can remain intact on the peritoneum.

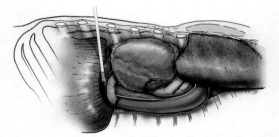

Fig. 5. A cuff of the diaphragm is created on the mediastinum over the aorta and esophagus. This cuff is created for an edge to suture the diaphragm patch medially to prevent herniation. (© 2020 Baylor College of Medicine.)

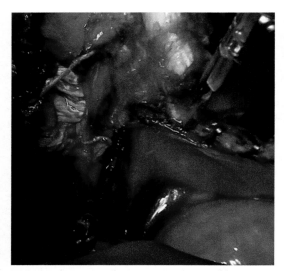

Fig. 6. The medial diaphragm is transected with cautery while applying clips to the medial edge to prevent bleeding.

approach enables rolling the disease toward the abdomen while removing it from the mediastinum until the diaphragm is exposed. Removal of bulky disease from the anterior and posterior chest wall resections helps visualize this area. At this point, the entire parietal pleurectomy is completed unless the pericardium requires resection. Disease can remain on the pericardium until after the visceral decortication is completed.

Step 6: Visceral Decortication

The goal of the visceral decortication is to remove all tumor, to expand the trapped lung, and to minimize air leaks. Intermittent inflation or the addition of positive pressure helps define the appropriate plane; however, continuous ventilation is associated with loss of tidal volume and increased blood

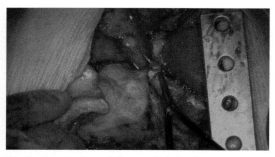

Fig. 7. Transection of the medial diaphragm requires prevention of tension on the phrenic veins that are at risk for avulsion injury, which can tear along the IVC into the abdomen.

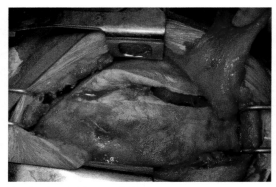

Fig. 8. The thickness of the tumor can prevent exposure to parts of the mediastinum. Starting the decortication by debulking the tumor can assist with exposure to the critical structures.

loss. This dissection can be tedious and add significant time compared with an EPP.

The visceral decortication is started by inflating the lungs and cutting through the tumor with a knife to the pulmonary parenchyma. The lung tissue bubbles when the appropriate plane is reached. With gentle retraction of the parenchyma with 1 hand covered by laparotomy pad, the lung is separated from the visceral pleura with a combination of blunt and sharp dissection (Fig. 10). Often, the disease is densely attached to corners such as the left upper lobe lingula; wedge resections may be necessary for a complete resection. The dissection is completed when the visceral pleurectomy reaches the hilum and the prior parietal pleurectomy. As noted previously, a complete hilar exposure during the parietal pleurectomy

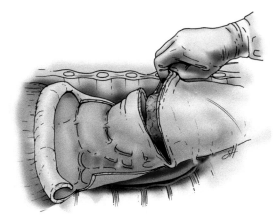

Fig. 9. As an alternative to exposure of the inferior mediastinum and the diaphragm, visceral decortication along the diaphragmatic surface of the lung provides access to the inferior pulmonary vein. (© 2020 Baylor College of Medicine.)

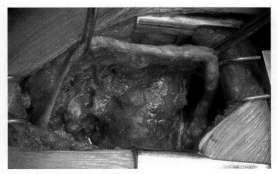

Fig. 10. The visceral decortication separates the pleura from the parenchyma in a distinct plane, but one that involves blood vessels. Intermittent insufflation of the lung can help identify this plane.

greatly facilitates the completion of the visceral pleurectomy.

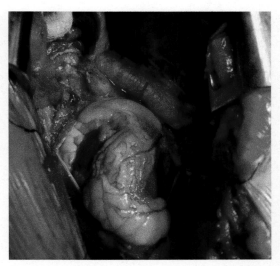

Fig. 11. Pericardiectomy extends from the confluence of the diaphragm inferiorly to the great vessels superiorly. The anterior incision is based on the location of invasive disease. Frozen section of the pericardium helps determine the location for the anterior transection. The posterior incision above the pulmonary veins is approached from inside the pericardium.

Step 7: Pericardial Resection

During the anterior parietal dissection, the pleura is resected off the fibrous pericardium. At the point at which the pleura cannot be peeled off the pericardium, it is opened. As the anterior pericardium is opened, stay sutures are placed and tied to the anterior incision to prevent retraction of the pericardium to the contralateral side. The pericardiectomy is extended superiorly to the great vessels and inferiorly to the diaphragm. The pericardium with disease is lifted to expose the pulmonary veins. From an intrapericardial approach, it is transected above the veins to complete the most posterior portion of the dissection. Once transected, the pericardium is lifted to expose the extrapericardial veins, which connects this dissection to the previous hilar dissections (**Fig. 11**). The margins are sent for frozen section analysis to determine whether more pericardial resection is required. At this point in the operation, all of the disease should be removed.

Step 8: Lymph Node Dissection, Thoracic Duct Ligation, and Betadine Scrub

Lymph node dissection is performed for staging information with the same stations developed for lung cancer; however, the dissections are more extensive with MPM. On the right, levels 4R, 7, 8R, 9R, 10R, and 11R are performed. On the left, levels 5, 6, 7, 8R, 9R, 10R, and 11R are performed. In addition, the internal mammary, the pericardial fat pad, diaphragmatic nodes, and posterior intercostal lymph nodes are removed. These dissections can be performed at the completion of the operation; however, performing throughout the operation as noted previously corresponds to the appropriate dissections.

Given the extensive dissection along the mediastinum, thoracic duct ligation is often performed for right-sided operations. The duct is tied with 0 silk sutures as low as possible near the diaphragm. This ligation is performed before reconstruction of the diaphragm. Alternatively, cream with methylene blue is injected into the nasogastric tube. Leaks are assessed and, if not present, the thoracic duct does not require ligation. This approach is appropriate for both left-sided and right-sided operations.

Povidone-iodine is administered to the intrathoracic cavity after complete resection and before reconstruction of the diaphragm and pericardium. Lang-Lazdunski and colleagues[12] reported that hyperthermic heated povidone-iodine compared favorably with other intraoperative adjuncts. Sterile water is mixed with 10% povidone-iodine at 40°C to 41°C for 5 minutes. Other intraoperative therapies are discussed in another article in this issue.

Step 9: Diaphragm Reconstruction

The diaphragm is reconstructed with a nonabsorbable patch that is usually 1-mm to 2-mm polytetrafluoroethylene (PTFE). The diaphragm patch is placed in the native position at the eighth intercostal space anteriorly, ninth intercostal space laterally, and 10th intercostal space posteriorly (**Fig. 12**). However, given that postoperative complications may occur with space management, the diaphragm can be placed 1 to 2 interspaces higher if the lung has been chronically trapped and is not likely to fully expand. With a high-volume tumor or chronic effusion with an atelectatic lung, placement of the diaphragm along the eighth intercostal space from anterior to posterior may prevent a chronic space.

The reconstruction is started by placing no. 2 Vicryl sutures from under the chosen rib, through the diaphragm patch as a vertical mattress corresponding with the size of the rib (about 1 cm), and back through the chest wall above the same rib. The vertical mattress in the patch is placed through the abdominal side of the patch so that the free edge is directed toward the thoracic cavity. Multiple sutures from anterior to posterior along the ribs to the level of the erector spinae muscles are inserted. Once the sutures in the lateral diaphragm are inserted, they are tied to the ribs. After these are tied, the medial sutures set the size and tautness of the patch. Anteriorly, part of the muscular diaphragm is often present and the patch is sewn to the muscle between the chest wall and the pericardium. Next, the patch is sewn to the confluence of the diaphragm and pericardium with 0-Prolene interrupted sutures. The diaphragm is reconstructed before the pericardium because these sutures are much easier to place without the pericardial patch. The medial border is continued along the diaphragm cuff across the aorta and the esophagus (see **Fig. 12**). Without a cuff, the mediastinal tissue does not have the strength for suture placement that prevents medial herniation of the abdominal viscera. On the right, the patch must not compromise the IVC. The final part of the reconstruction closes the area over the vertebral bodies between the cuff and the posterior rib sutures. This area is tacked to the vertebral bodies with a laparoscopic 5-mm tacking device. The vertical mattress sutures are placed with the edge toward the thoracic cavity so that the free edge of the patch covers this area and can be tacked in multiple places.

Step 10: Pericardial Reconstruction

If the pericardium was resected, it is reconstructed at this point. The patch consists of 0.1-mm PTFE sewn circumferentially to the pericardium with 2-0 Prolene sutures (**Fig. 13**). Vicryl mesh is an alternative that may decrease postoperative pericarditis. The superior pericardium over the great vessels does not need to be closed. The inferior pericardium is sewn to the confluence of the diaphragm and pericardium directly to the diaphragm patch (**Fig. 14**). The pericardial reconstruction prevents herniation and torsion. The patch must be loose enough to prevent restriction. It is fenestrated to prevent tamponade. Some surgeons avoid reconstruction to prevent risk of infection and rely on the lung to prevent cardiac herniation.

OUTCOMES AND COMPARISON WITH EXTRAPLEURAL PNEUMONECTOMY

ePD versus EPP has never undergone direct comparison; however, ePD has become the preferred operation at many institutions.[13] The complication rates were assessed by the Mesothelioma and Radical Surgery (MARS 1) trial, a meta-analysis comparing ePD with EPP, and improvement in patient management contribute to this change.[1,14–16]

A meta-analysis of 19 studies report that the 30-day mortality for ePD versus EPP was significantly lower at 1.7% versus 4.5%.[16] Prior studies are consistent with the findings showing a lower

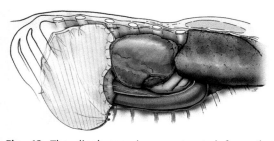

Fig. 12. The diaphragm is reconstructed from the eighth intercostal space anteriorly, ninth intercostal space laterally, and 10th intercostal space posteriorly. If the lung is unlikely to fill this space from chronic entrapment, then the diaphragm patch can be placed 1 to 2 interspaces higher. The medial patch is sewn to the confluence of the pericardium and a cuff of native diaphragm over the esophagus and the aorta. (© 2020 Baylor College of Medicine.)

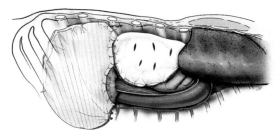

Fig. 13. The pericardial patch consists of 0.1-mm thick PTFE sewn circumferentially to the pericardium with surgical sutures. The patch must be loose enough to prevent restriction and fenestrated to prevent tamponade. (© 2020 Baylor College of Medicine.)

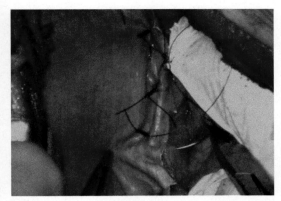

Fig. 14. The pericardial patch is sewn directly to the confluence of the diaphragm and pericardium through the diaphragm patch. This reconstruction is easiest when the diaphragm patch is placed first.

mortality with ePD compared with EPP.[13,17,18] Sharkey and colleagues[13] reported that patients undergoing ePD were older (65 vs 57 years old) with lower performance status (35.4% vs 46.3% with ≥1), but still had a mortality after ePD at 90 days that was lower than patients undergoing EPP.

Based on the IASLC mesothelioma database, the median overall survival (OS) after pleurectomy and decortication (PD) was 23, 20, 19, and 15 months for stage I, II, III, IV, respectively.[19] Whether the operation was a PD or ePD was uncertain. From that dataset, the median OS after EPP was 40, 23, 16, and 12 months for stage I, II, III, IV, respectively. Based on the meta-analysis, the OS after ePD versus EPP was longer in 47% and 53%, respectively. They did acknowledge that significant heterogeneity in the results exists; therefore, these groups may not be comparable. Sharkey and colleagues[13] reported no difference in the OS between the operations. On a subgroup analysis, they noted a higher OS after ePD for patients more than 65 years old. With a lower mortality with ePD, uncertain OS advantage with EPP, and better outcomes in old and frail patients, ePD has become more common at most mesothelioma centers.

The role of surgery was questioned in the MARS 1 trial, in which 24 patients were enrolled over 3 years in the EPP arm, of whom 16 underwent an EPP.[14] The feasibility of enrolling 50 patients in 1 year was the primary outcome, which was not met. Despite the low accrual and lack of power, they concluded that EPP is of no benefit and possibly causes harm. To answer this question and draw this conclusion, the trial would have required enrolling 670 patients.[20] At present, the MARS 2 (a feasibility study comparing [extended] pleurectomy decortication versus no pleurectomy and decortication in patients with malignant pleural mesothelioma) is nearing accrual. Patients will receive 2 cycles of neoadjuvant cisplatin and pemetrexed then will be randomized to receive lung-sparing surgery followed by 4 more cycles of chemotherapy versus chemotherapy alone. It is hoped that this trial will help clarify the role of ePD in MPM.

SUMMARY

With lower perioperative mortality, similar long-term survival, and better tolerance in patients with lower performance status, ePD has become the preferred operation rather than EPP despite lack of a direct comparison. As ePD has become more popular, international collaboration is underway to create surgical guidelines based on collection of operative data. It is hoped that these efforts will improve the safety and standardization of this operation. Although not the focus of this article, ePD is a component of multimodality strategies that include chemotherapeutics and radiotherapy after lung preservation.

ePD is a difficult operation performed for the surgical resection of MPM that can achieve a macroscopic complete resection with preservation of the lung. The chest anatomy viewed from the extrapleural planes is an infrequent approach for most surgeons. Meticulous surgical technique with multiple long steps is required for patients to have a good outcome.

CLINICS CARE POINTS

- ePD is a lung-sparing surgery that indicates a visceral and parietal pleurectomy with the resection of the diaphragm and/or pericardium.
- The goal of curative surgical resection is to achieve a macroscopic complete resection, which may be accomplished by ePD.
- The goal of the visceral decortication is to remove all tumor, to expand the trapped lung, and to minimize air leaks.
- Routine resection of the diaphragm is unnecessary, and preservation of the muscular diaphragm with primary closure is feasible for disease that does not invade, or minimally invades, the muscular diaphragm.
- Creation of a cuff of diaphragm along the mediastinum over the aorta and esophagus helps reconstruct the diaphragm patch and prevent herniation.
- The visceral decortication with debulking of large tumors can be performed before a

complete parietal pleurectomy to safely approach the mediastinum and hilum.

- Compared with EPP, ePD has a lower perioperative mortality, similar long-term survival, and better tolerance in patients with lower performance status. ePD has become the preferred operation in many centers despite lack of a direct comparison.
- Preoperative assessment includes PFTs with DLco, VQ scans, echocardiography, and often cardiology consultation.
- Preoperative staging includes imaging with CT, PET, and occasionally MRI, as well as invasive biopsies with diagnostic laparoscopy, mediastinoscopy, and ipsilateral and contralateral VATS biopsies as needed.

ACKNOWLEDGMENTS

The author would like to thank Scott C. Holmes, CMI, a member of the Michael E. DeBakey Department of Surgery at Baylor College of Medicine, for his graphic assistance during the preparation of this article.

DISCLOSURE

The author has nothing to disclose.

REFERENCES

1. Bueno R, Opitz I, Taskforce IM. Surgery in malignant pleural mesothelioma. J Thorac Oncol 2018;13(11): 1638–54.
2. Baas P, et al. Malignant pleural mesothelioma: ESMO clinical practice guidelines for diagnosis, treatment and follow-up. Ann Oncol 2015;26(Suppl 5):v31–9.
3. Ettinger DS, et al. NCCN guidelines insights: malignant pleural mesothelioma, version 3.2016. J Natl Compr Canc Netw 2016;14(7):825–36.
4. Kindler HL, et al. Treatment of malignant pleural mesothelioma: american society of clinical oncology clinical practice guideline. J Clin Oncol 2018; 36(13):1343–73.
5. Rice D, et al. Recommendations for uniform definitions of surgical techniques for malignant pleural mesothelioma: a consensus report of the international association for the study of lung cancer international staging committee and the international mesothelioma interest group. J Thorac Oncol 2011; 6(8):1304–12.
6. Friedberg JS, et al. A proposed system toward standardizing surgical-based treatments for malignant pleural mesothelioma, from the joint national cancer institute-international association for the study of lung cancer-mesothelioma applied research foundation taskforce. J Thorac Oncol 2019;14(8):1343–53.
7. Husain AN, et al. Guidelines for pathologic diagnosis of malignant mesothelioma: 2012 update of the consensus statement from the International Mesothelioma Interest Group. Arch Pathol Lab Med 2013;137(5):647–67.
8. Paintal A, et al. The diagnosis of malignant mesothelioma in effusion cytology: a reappraisal and results of a multi-institution survey. Cancer Cytopathol 2013; 121(12):703–7.
9. Pass H, et al. The IASLC mesothelioma staging project: improving staging of a rare disease through international participation. J Thorac Oncol 2016; 11(12):2082–8.
10. Rusch VW, et al. A multicenter study of volumetric computed tomography for staging malignant pleural mesothelioma. Ann Thorac Surg 2016;102(4): 1059–66.
11. Rice DC, et al. Extended surgical staging for potentially resectable malignant pleural mesothelioma. Ann Thorac Surg 2005;80(6):1988–92 [discussion: 1992–3].
12. Lang-Lazdunski L, et al. Pleurectomy/decortication, hyperthermic pleural lavage with povidone-iodine followed by adjuvant chemotherapy in patients with malignant pleural mesothelioma. J Thorac Oncol 2011;6(10):1746–52.
13. Sharkey AJ, et al. The effects of an intentional transition from extrapleural pneumonectomy to extended pleurectomy/decortication. Eur J Cardiothorac Surg 2016;49(6):1632–41.
14. Treasure T, et al. Extra-pleural pneumonectomy versus no extra-pleural pneumonectomy for patients with malignant pleural mesothelioma: clinical outcomes of the Mesothelioma and Radical Surgery (MARS) randomised feasibility study. Lancet Oncol 2011;12(8):763–72.
15. Kostron A, et al. Propensity matched comparison of extrapleural pneumonectomy and pleurectomy/ decortication for mesothelioma patients. Interact Cardiovasc Thorac Surg 2017;24(5):740–6.
16. Taioli E, Wolf AS, Flores RM. Meta-analysis of survival after pleurectomy decortication versus extrapleural pneumonectomy in mesothelioma. Ann Thorac Surg 2015;99(2):472–80.
17. Cao C, et al. A systematic review and meta-analysis of surgical treatments for malignant pleural mesothelioma. Lung Cancer 2014;83(2):240–5.
18. Cao CQ, et al. A systematic review of extrapleural pneumonectomy for malignant pleural mesothelioma. J Thorac Oncol 2010;5(10):1692–703.
19. Rusch VW, et al. Initial analysis of the international association for the study of lung cancer mesothelioma database. J Thorac Oncol 2012;7(11):1631–9.
20. Weder W, et al. The MARS feasibility trial: conclusions not supported by data. Lancet Oncol 2011; 12(12):1093–4 [author reply: 1094–5].

The Role of Extrapleural Pneumonectomy in Malignant Pleural Mesothelioma

Laura L. Donahoe, MD, MSc, FRCSC[a], Marc de Perrot, MD, MSc, FRCSC[b],*

KEYWORDS

- Mesothelioma • Extrapleural pneumonectomy • Surgery • Multimodality therapy

KEY POINTS

- Although there is no standard-of-care for surgical management of mesothelioma, all patients with early stage should be considered for macroscopic complete resection.
- Extrapleural pneumonectomy should be considered as part of multimodal therapy for epithelioid mesothelioma with diffuse pleural involvement and invasion of the lung parenchyma.
- A minority of patients with mesothelioma are candidates for extrapleural pneumonectomy, yet this subset of patients can derive long-term benefit.

BACKGROUND

Malignant pleural mesothelioma (MPM) continues to be a worldwide health concern due to industrial and environmental exposure to asbestos.[1] Despite extensive research worldwide, the prognosis remains poor with median survivals ranging between 12.3 and 18.8 months in large randomized clinical trials.[2–5] The poor prognosis is often due to delayed diagnosis and the rapid progression of the disease once an invasive component is present on histologic examination. The recent identification of some gene alterations, such as BRCA1-associated protein 1 loss and CDKN2A (p16) homozygous deletion could potentially provide an opportunity to detect the mesothelioma in an in situ or preinvasive phase, which may change the treatment paradigm by intervening earlier and more effectively in the future.[6]

Currently, the standard-of-care for MPM is limited to chemotherapy with cisplatin-pemetrexed and possibly bevacizumab for patients who are not surgical candidates.[2,4,5] There is no recognized standard-of-care for patients who are surgical candidates and therefore these patients should be included into clinical trials investigating multimodal approaches as often as possible. Recent breakthroughs in immunotherapy could potentially offer new opportunities to improve outcome in this devastating disease. However, despite the carcinogenic impact of asbestos, single-agent immunotherapy so far had limited benefit in mesothelioma.[7] A large randomized double-blinded trial with tremelimumab, a cytotoxic-T-lymphocyte-associated antigen 4 monoclonal antibody, across 19 countries in second- and third-line therapy for mesothelioma was negative compared with best supportive care.[8] Double-agent immunotherapy offers more promising results, but large randomized trials are not yet available in mesothelioma.[9,10] Preclinical work demonstrates that combining immunotherapy with conventional therapy could provide the best approach to treat mesothelioma.[11,12] A large randomized trial comparing cisplatin-pemetrexed with or without pembrolizumab for

a Division of Thoracic Surgery, Toronto General Hospital, Princess Margaret Cancer Center, University Health Network, Toronto, Canada; b Mesothelioma Program, Division of Thoracic Surgery, University Health Network, Princess Margaret Cancer Center, Toronto General Hospital, 9N-961, Toronto, Ontario M5G 2C4, Canada
* Corresponding author.
E-mail address: Marc.deperrot@uhn.ca

first-line therapy in nonsurgical patients is thus ongoing in Canada, France, and Italy. In early-stage disease, studies are investigating the role of immunotherapy and chemo-immunotherapy in combination with surgery. We are also conducting a phase I clinical trial with oligofractionated radiation before surgery (Surgery for Mesothelioma After Radiation Therapy Using Extensive Pleural Resection [SMARTER] trial) to use this approach as a platform for immunotherapy.

The role of surgery in mesothelioma is controversial because of the inability to do a complete resection (R0) in the context of disseminated tumor in the pleural cavity. However, subgroup analysis in large surgical series demonstrate that selected patients can potentially benefit from radical surgery with median survival greater than 3 years.[13] A propensity score match analysis from the National Cancer Database also demonstrated that radical surgery provided a small but overall significant survival benefit, particularly in epithelioid MPM.[14] The general consensus among surgeons, medical oncologists, and radiation oncologists specialized in mesothelioma is that complete macroscopic resection (MCR) can provide benefit in selected patients as long as it is performed as part of a multidisciplinary protocol.[15,16]

SURGICAL OPTIONS

The 2 main surgical options for aggressive management of MPM are extrapleural pneumonectomy (EPP) and extended pleurectomy-decortication (EPD). There is much debate in the literature regarding the merits and drawbacks of both techniques, and a move away from performing EPP has occurred because of concerns about the peri- and postoperative morbidity.[17] EPD is a lesser surgery, in which the lung is preserved while attempting to remove most of the visceral and parietal pleural, and generally still involves partial resection and reconstruction of the diaphragm or pericardium. The main advantage of EPD is the decreased morbidity associated with preserving the lung, which may result in an improved ability to complete adjuvant treatment due to better physiologic reserve postoperatively. Disadvantages of this technique compared with EPP include the fact that it is nonstandardized, presents issues when considering the use of adjuvant radiation therapy, and is less likely to result in an R1 resection. These limitations are recognized and being addressed to facilitate comparison between surgical series.[18]

Currently, direct comparison between EPP and EPD is limited by the lack of prospective clinical trials comparing both surgical options. Indirect comparison is difficult as EPP is generally done for more advanced disease and EPD is more frequently used in patients with early-stage disease.[19] Registry studies are also difficult to interpret as EPP is done more frequently in centers with limited mesothelioma activity with high operative mortality, whereas EPD has been concentrated in a few large US centers with mesothelioma expertise.[20] The SEER database does suggest that the most important parameter to improve survival is the ability to receive treatment in expert mesothelioma centers, independently of the type of surgery.[21]

EXTRAPLEURAL PNEUMONECTOMY

The first large series of EPP for mesothelioma was published in 1976, and described 29 patients who underwent surgery for mesothelioma.[22] Interestingly, some of the findings of the study still hold true today: survival after EPP is worse for biphasic and sarcomatoid subtypes, and EPP should not be used as a single-modality treatment due to the poor overall survival.[22,23] EPP became more frequently performed after the publication from Rusch and colleagues[24] in 2001 demonstrating the potential benefit of adjuvant high-dose hemithoracic radiation after EPP on local control. They observed an in-field recurrence rate of only 13% after the administration of 54 Gy in 30 fractions over 6 weeks using 3D conformal radiation therapy. The group in the MD Anderson Cancer center introduced the use of intensity modality radiation therapy (IMRT) after EPP for mesothelioma, confirming the excellent local control with high-dose hemithoracic radiation post-EPP.[25] IMRT was particularly helpful to optimize the delivery of radiation in the lower chest along the lumbar spine where the risk of local failure was greatest.[25–27] Despite initial concerns about the use of IMRT after EPP, multiple studies have now confirmed the safety of high-dose hemithoracic IMRT after EPP when strict constraints are applied to the contralateral lung.[28]

Several large (greater than 40 patients) prospective single-arm phase 2 clinical trials were performed using induction chemotherapy to reduce the risk of distant relapse followed by EPP and adjuvant hemithoracic radiation.[29–34] The overall median survival in most of these studies ranged between 15.5 and 22.4 months as an intention-to-treat analysis (**Table 1**). The survival of patients who completed all 3 modalities was improved, ranging between 29.1 and 39.4 months, but a large number of patients dropped out, demonstrating the difficulty to perform EPP in a multimodality

Table 1
Prospective clinical trials with chemotherapy-extrapleural pneumonectomy-hemithoracic radiation for malignant pleural mesothelioma

First Author, Year	Patients Starting Chemotherapy	Patients Completing Radiation Therapy	Survival Intention-to-Treat (mo)	Survival Treatment Completed (mo)
Weder et al,[29] 2007	61	36 (59%)	19.8	NS
Krug et al,[30] 2009	77	40 (52%)	16.8	29.1
Van Schil et al,[31] 2010	59	37 (63%)	18.4	33
Federico et al,[32] 2013	54	22 (41%)	15.5	NS
Hasegawa et al,[33] 2016	42	17 (40%)	19.9	39.4
Frick et al,[34] 2019	97	47 (48%)	22.4	33.2

Abbreviations: mo, months; NS, not specified.

therapy setting with 3 to 4 cycles of chemotherapy and 6 weeks of radiation.

The multicenter phase II US trial showed that the benefit of hemithoracic radiation after EPP was independent of the response to induction chemotherapy.[30] Indeed, patients who responded to induction chemotherapy had a median survival of 26 months after EPP and 30 months after hemithoracic radiation. In sharp contrast, patients who presented with stable or progression of disease on chemotherapy had a median survival of only 17 months after EPP, whereas it was 28 months after hemithoracic radiation. This observation emphasizes the intrinsic benefit of EPP and hemithoracic radiation independently of chemotherapy. The 2-year survival of patients who completed the trimodality therapy in this large multicenter US trial reached 61%, a dramatic improvement over the 2-year survival of 33% after EPP alone in the multicenter phase II trial performed by the Lung Cancer Study Group between 1985 and 1988.[30,35]

The Mesothelioma and Radical Surgery trial is the only randomized trial in surgery for mesothelioma.[36] It was designed as a feasibility study to address whether a large randomized trial could be performed to determine the benefit of EPP in mesothelioma or lack thereof. The study could not recruit an adequate number of patients to proceed to a large randomized trial demonstrating the difficulty to randomize patients to a surgical arm against a nonsurgical arm in MPM. Despite the limited accrual, the study did demonstrate worse outcome in patients undergoing EPP, which was due in large part to the high operative mortality in this small sample size, highlighting the importance of having expert centers only performing this surgery.[37]

EVIDENCE FOR EXTRAPLEURAL PNEUMONECTOMY

Several retrospective analyses have been performed to compare EPP to EPD, but surgeons have an inherent tendency to favor 1 option over the other based on their personal experience and center expertise.[38] Conceptually, EPD would be more appropriate for patients with limited bulk disease, whereas EPP would be better for patients with locally advanced disease. EPD can also be performed in locally advanced disease, particularly in epithelioid tumors (**Fig. 1**). However, the morbidity of this approach for locally advanced disease remains high as it requires several hours to decorticate the lungs with important blood loss and risk of prolonged air leaks and potential pleural space complications postoperatively. Increasing evidence demonstrates that the extent of visceral pleural involvement, the degree of lung parenchyma invasion, and the presence of lymph node involvement can increase the risk of lung recurrence and poor outcome after EPD, supporting the concept that EPP may be more beneficial in patients with extensive pleural involvement and diffuse invasion of the lung parenchyma.[39,40] Boutin and colleagues[40] observed that MPM with nonspecific inflammatory visceral lesions and visceral nodules smaller than 5 mm during thoracoscopy were associated with good prognosis, reaching a median survival of 28 months. This observation was confirmed by Rusch and Venkatraman,[41] who observed a median survival of 27 months in the presence of scattered pleural involvement compared with 12 months in the presence of confluent visceral pleural disease. In patients undergoing EPD, the absence of invasion of the visceral pleura beyond

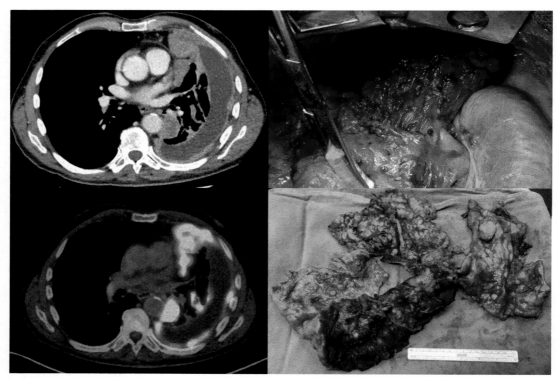

Fig. 1. EPD can be performed in patients with locally advanced mesothelioma. Direct comparison between EPD and EPP has never been performed. Both options have advantages and limitations and are not exclusive. EPD and EPP should be part of prospective clinical trials with predefined multimodality approach and clear definition of the type of surgery performed.

the elastic lamina can be associated with prolonged disease-free survival of up to 80% at 3 years, whereas invasion in the lung parenchyma is associated with a disease-free survival of less than 18 months.[39] A recent study also demonstrated that lymphangitic recurrences in the lung parenchyma was frequent, occurring in up to 39% of the patients after EPD, and was associated with worse outcome.[42] These observations emphasize the potential limitation of EPD in the presence of extensive lung involvement and support the potential value of EPP in this context.

Our experience in Toronto has demonstrated that careful evaluation and adequate patient selection can be associated with good outcome after EPP.[43] EPP does require extremely meticulous postoperative care with attention to details to prevent complications. Complications after EPP carry a major risk of spiraling down as the patients have minimal reserve. These complications can then lead to early mortality or long-term frailty with worse survival.

In our practice, we generally prefer EPP over EPD whenever the physiologic status of the patients is adequate, optimal postoperative care

can be provided, and other therapeutic modalities can be safely administered. The most notable exception is in the presence of minimal visceral pleural disease where preserving the lung can provide good long-term results with EPD. We do believe, however, that the difference between EPP and EPD is limited as long as an MCR is performed. Hence, the emphasis should not so much focus on the type of surgery but rather on the ability to deliver and complete a predefined multimodality approach in the context of an MCR. We need to have well-designed prospective clinical trials to be able to assess the values of MCR in the context of a multimodality approach. These trials should prospectively collect data and report the intention-to-treat outcome, which are currently lacking in many series of EPD.

It is becoming increasingly evident that the subtypes of epithelioid mesothelioma and the different genetic alterations in mesothelioma can affect survival.[44,45] Hence, these factors need to be taken into consideration to understand the impact of surgery and multimodality approach on outcome. Bilecz and colleagues[44] recently reported that tubulopapillary and microcystic epithelioid mesothelioma were associated with a median survival of nearly 3 years and 5-year survival of 40% after multimodality therapy, whereas solid and trabecular epithelioid mesothelioma were associated with median survival of less than 2 years and 5-year survival of less than 20% after multimodality therapy. Interestingly, the different epithelioid subtypes did not affect survival in patients treated with chemotherapy and best supportive care, suggesting that the epithelioid subtypes are particularly important in early-stage disease amenable to surgery.

EXTRAPLEURAL PNEUMONECTOMY AND RADIATION THERAPY

Based on the impressive local control obtained with high-dose hemithoracic radiation after EPP, we developed a new protocol with hemithoracic radiation before surgery that was named Surgery for Mesothelioma After Radiation Therapy (SMART) to be able to deliver optimal radiation to the whole tumor bed before resection. The importance of radiation in the treatment of mesothelioma was supported by in vitro and in vivo experiments demonstrating that mesothelioma cell lines were more sensitive to radiation than non-small cell lung cancer cell lines.[46,47] Palliative radiation is also successful in controlling pain or mediastinal invasion in the context of locally advanced mesothelioma.[26] The SMART protocol includes a short course of hypofractionated radiation (25–30 Gy) delivered in 5 daily fractions over 1 week followed by surgery a week later. The short time frame between radiation and surgery was chosen to limit the risk of radiation-induced pneumonitis. The goal of the radiation was to sterilize the tumor edges and prevent seeding to the peritoneal, pericardial, and contralateral pleural cavities.

Our initial experience with a seamless phase I–II trial demonstrated the safety of this protocol with 25 patients.[48] We observed that survival was significantly better in epithelioid than in biphasic MPM and therefore have subsequently limited the trial to epithelioid mesothelioma. The rate of grade 3 and 4 postoperative complications was 39%, which was similar to our previous experience with induction chemotherapy.[49] Noteworthy, patients undergoing EPP after radiation required significantly less blood transfusions than after induction chemotherapy, thus potentially limiting the overall morbidity of this treatment compared with preoperative chemotherapy.[49] The SMART treatment is also short in duration compared with the trimodality approach, which provides benefit in patients traveling long distances. Once patients recover from the radiation and surgery, they can enjoy a lifestyle similar to patients undergoing pneumonectomy for other types of malignancy.

We currently have treated more than 120 patients with this protocol. The updated results with 110 patients were presented in 2018 at the International Mesothelioma Interest Group meeting in Ottawa. At the time, 85 treatment-naive patients were treated on protocol for cT1-3N0 MPM and 25 patients were treated off protocol due to predominantly N2 or T4 disease (n = 12), previous chemotherapy (n = 5), and synchronous tumors (n = 5). The 30- and 90-day mortality rates were 0.9% and 3.6%, respectively, with a median survival of 27.3 months for the whole cohort and no significant difference between patients treated on and off protocol. Most patients had T3 and T4 tumors with positive nodal disease on final pathology. The best outcome was achieved in patients with node-negative epithelioid mesothelioma. Chemotherapy was initially planned for patients with N2 disease on final pathology, but the difficulty to deliver chemotherapy within an adequate timeframe after EPP led us to modify the protocol and only administer chemotherapy at the time of recurrence.[50]

PATIENT SELECTION FOR SURGERY FOR MESOTHELIOMA AFTER RADIATION THERAPY

Our selection process for SMART is guided by the histologic type of mesothelioma, staging, local extent of disease, and physiologic workup. All our patients must have a histologic confirmation of mesothelioma. Biopsies performed outside our institution are reviewed by our pathologists and a subtypes is determined if possible. Currently, all our patients have BRCA1-associated protein 1 loss and p16 deletion tested. Patients with sarcomatoid and biphasic mesothelioma are typically excluded from the SMART approach. The only exceptions have been young patients with clinical stage I biphasic mesothelioma, which we have very occasionally treated with a SMART approach. However, despite this initial selection process, we do see biphasic disease in the final pathology of the EPP specimen in more than 20% of the patients who were deemed epithelioid on the preoperative biopsy.

Patients are staged with a computed tomography (CT) scan of the chest-abdomen and pelvis, PET-CT scan, and brain MRI. Mediastinal and hilar lymph nodes staging are then performed with endobrochial ultrasound (EBUS). All our imaging is performed within 6 weeks of the start of radiation and generally after pleurodesis to ensure that the pleural effusion does not interfere with the evaluation of the CT scan and the delivery of radiation as the accumulation of pleural fluid could affect the planning CT. The patient's performance status is also carefully evaluated, as is the severity of symptoms. The presence and location of chest pain and the need for daily opioid medications are recorded. Opioid-dependent chest pain is a worrisome sign for the ability to perform an EPP due to chest wall invasion and generally a contraindication to SMART.

The ability to complete an EPP is then decided based on the CT scan. The areas that are reviewed in details include the chest wall, the thoracic inlet, the mediastinum, the mainstem bronchus (to ensure that there is adequate length to staple it), the esophagus, the aorta, the pericardium, and the diaphragm. The overall bulk of disease is also assessed as we found that the total tumor thickness was a good correlate to the tumor volume and an independent predictor of survival. The diaphragmatic tumor thickness is also assessed on the sagittal and coronal CT reconstructions with 3-mm slices.[51] Diffuse diaphragmatic tumor thickness with total thickness greater than 4 cm by adding the measurement of 3 separate sites was associated with poor prognosis in our experience (**Fig. 2**). The poorer outcome with greater diaphragmatic thickness may be related to the difficulty to achieve an MCR in the posterior diaphragmatic sulcus or from preferential lymphatic drainage into the upper abdomen. Local chest wall extensions are not necessarily a contraindication to SMART as the chest wall can be resected en bloc with the EPP specimen (**Fig. 3**). Patients with N2 disease are not candidates for EPP. However, we have considered proceeding with SMART off protocol in younger patients with other favorable prognostic factors and only 1 site of low bulk N2 disease. Noteworthy, the biopsy from EBUS or endoscopic ultrasound (EUS) can accidently be contaminated by the primary tumor itself and be false positive. We have observed this in a young patient after EUS who was then treated with SMART off protocol, confirming the negative nodal status.

All patients being considered for EPP will have a physiologic workup with a full set of pulmonary function tests (PFTs), including diffusing capacity of lung for carbon monoxide (D_{LCO}), a ventilation-perfusion (VQ) lung scan and an echocardiogram. Many patients have a restrictive pattern on PFTs. Hence, D_{LCO} is the best parameter to rule out parenchymal lung disease. We typically would consider a D_{LCO} at baseline of less than 60% and a predicted postoperative D_{LCO} of less than 45% as a contraindication for EPP. The VQ scan often shows a perfusion of around 30% in the affected

lung in the absence of residual pleural effusion. Patients with lung perfusion of less than 20% are closely assessed, but is not be a contraindication for a SMART approach by itself. Using a combination of clinical assessment, CT scan, and VQ scan to determine the feasibility of EPP has allowed us to reduce our rate of exploratory thoracotomy to zero in patients treated with the SMART protocol, despite operating on 26% of the patients who we evaluated in clinic, including tumors with volume up to 3539 cm^3.[51]

Cardiac workup is also performed for all patients being considered for EPP. Echocardiography is always done to rule out pulmonary hypertension, left ventricular dysfunction, and valvular abnormalities. The echocardiogram also allows us to rule out pericardial effusion and intrapericardial extension of the tumor. In the presence of a normal echocardiogram, no further cardiac investigations are performed with the exception of an exercise study in patients with a history of coronary disease or suspected angina.

INTRAOPERATIVE TECHNIQUE

EPP is performed on average 5 to 6 days after the end of radiation (range, 2–12 days). The resection begins with a large posterolateral incision and resection of the sixth rib to access the extrapleural plane. Resection of the fifth rib provides better access to the apex of the pleural cavity and is selected when we anticipate difficult dissection around the thoracic inlet. Using a combination of blunt and sharp extrapleural dissection, the tumor is mobilized off the chest wall along the extrapleural space. The dissection is then extended along the mediastinum to expose the pericardium, which is then opened anteriorly if invaded and dissected down to the diaphragm. The posterior pericardium is also opened behind the pulmonary veins, which allows a complete resection of the involved ipsilateral pericardium. The opened pericardium will facilitate exposure of the diaphragm anteriorly. Once the access becomes limited in the lower chest, a second thoracotomy is performed in the eighth intercostal space (**Fig. 4**). This second thoracotomy performed through the same skin incision allows increased visualization of the hemidiaphragm, especially posteriorly along the chest wall and in the area of the ipsilateral crus. The lower thoracotomy also allows improved visualization for sharp dissection of the diaphragm along the inferior vena cava on the right side and the esophagus on the left side. The thoracic duct is inspected, but not routinely ligated.

Once the specimen is removed, both the diaphragm and pericardium are reconstructed using

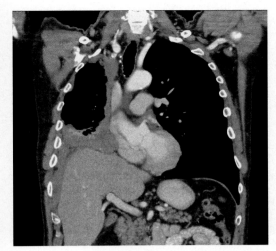

Fig. 2. EPP can be performed in the presence of large tumor volume. Retrospective review of our experience demonstrated that large diffuse diaphragmatic tumor thickness more specifically affected survival in the context of EPP after induction hemithoracic radiation.

Gore-Tex mesh (1 mm for diaphragm and 0.1 mm for pericardium). Two 1-mm Gore-Tex meshes are stapled together to have adequate length for the diaphragm. The diaphragmatic mesh is attached with interrupted stitches along the inferior part of the pericardium, the anterior cartilaginous part of the ribs, and the ninth intercostal space. Posteriorly, the mesh is also fixed by 1 stitch on the spine at the level of T8 or T9. Care is taken to avoid any impingement on the inferior vena cava on the right side or the esophagus and aorta on the left side. The pericardial mesh is attached by interrupted stitches to the anterior, inferior, and posterior part of the pericardium. The pericardial mesh is kept loose to avoid any cardiac constriction postoperatively. Several cuts are made in the pericardial mesh to avoid postoperative tamponade. If a large part of the pericardium is removed on the left side, we generally do not reconstruct the pericardium.

The bronchial stump is stapled and covered with the posterior pericardium, as previously described on the right and the left side.[52] The posterior pericardium is easily mobilized to cover the bronchial stump on the left. On the right side, the posterior pericardium is opened behind the right pulmonary veins and dissected off the wall of the left atrium along the oblique sinus. The pericardium is then freed from the pulmonary artery stump and the superior vena cava along the transverse sinus, allowing the posterior pericardium to be fully mobilized and attached to the structures behind the bronchial stump, such as the vagus nerve, the edge of the esophageal muscle, and the azygos vein (**Fig. 5**). This technique allows the bronchial stump to be "mediastinalized" and well protected. In our experience, the posterior pericardium could be used to cover the bronchial stump in more than 90% of the time. We observed 1 small bronchopleural fistula out of 120 patients undergoing the SMART approach using this technique.

POSTOPERATIVE MANAGEMENT

Postoperatively, patients are monitored in a step-down unit for 3 to 4 days after surgery. Some degree of hypotension is common, and usually managed with fluid replacement. Unlike the traditional dogma of fluid-restricting patients who have undergone pneumonectomy, in the early postoperative period after EPP judicious use of intravenous fluids is prescribed due to the large fluid shifts associated with the extensive dissection of this procedure. The chest tube remains in place for 3 to 4 days, predominantly to observe the character of the output and monitor for bleeding. Prophylactic antibiotics are continued until the chest tube is removed. Although a nasogastric tube is frequently used intraoperatively to aid in identifying the esophagus, it is removed before the completion of the procedure. Patients remain nil per os for the first 24 hours, then the diet is slowly advanced as bowel function returns.

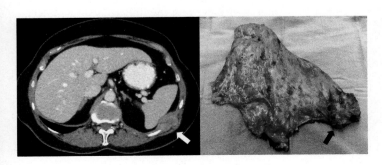

Fig. 3. EPP can be performed in combination with local chest wall resection. This patient had resection of ribs 11 and 12 (*arrow*) resected en bloc with the EPP.

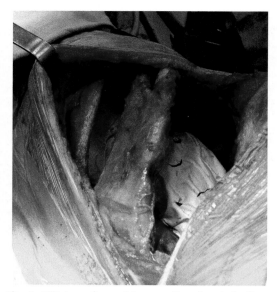

Fig. 4. EPP is performed by resecting the sixth rib to facilitate exposure and access the extrapleural plane. A second thoracotomy is performed in the eighth intercostal space to achieve complete resection of the diaphragm.

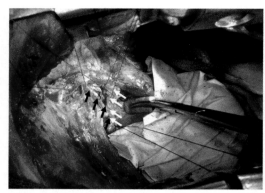

Fig. 5. The bronchus is closed with a stapler at about 1 cm from the carina. On the right side, the posterior pericardium is then freed from the left atrium and the pulmonary artery (*white arrows*) and sutured to the vagus nerve (*black arrows*) to "mediastinalize" the bronchial stump. This technique can be performed in the very vast majority of patients undergoing EPP and provide excellent protection.

Bloodwork is tested twice daily for the first few days. Electrolytes are actively replaced to limit the risk of atrial fibrillation. Prophylactic anticoagulation is started immediately postoperatively and maintained for 6 weeks after surgery as an outpatient after hospital discharge.

FUTURE PERSPECTIVE

Over the past decade, clinical and preclinical evidence have demonstrated that oligofractionated radiation characterized by a short course (2–5 fractions) of hypofractionated radiation can boost an antitumor immune response through the induction of type I interferon.[47,53] This effect has gained increasing interest over the past few years with the introduction of immune checkpoint blockade in clinical practice. The benefit of combining oligofractionated radiation with immune checkpoints has been particularly relevant in the context of metastatic disease.[54] Although the response rate has been variable, these studies have demonstrated that the combination of radiation and immunotherapy offers great potential.[55] One of the advantages of this new treatment paradigm is the ability to generate an immune activation by delivering a nonablative dose of radiation, thus limiting its toxicity.[47] Increasing evidence suggests that the antigen load is a key determinant of clinical response to immunotherapy and that even robust immune response may be clinically ineffective if

the tumor burden is high.[56] Hence, the combination of a short course of radiation to generate a specific antitumoral immune response followed by radical surgery to reduce the tumor antigen load to a minimal is a very promising concept.

Considering our results with the SMART approach and its impact on cytotoxic CD8+ T cells, which were shown to be an independent predictor of outcome after SMART, the concept of oligofractionated radiation followed by surgery could offer an ideal platform for immunotherapy in mesothelioma.[57] We have therefore designed a new clinical trial (the SMARTER trial). This trial is a phase I approach with increasing doses of nonablative oligofractionated radiation to the pleural space delivered in 3 fractions over 1 week to determine its safety in the context of EPD and its impact on the immune system (**Fig. 6**). Based on our preclinical experience and the literature, we estimate that a dose of radiation of 18 to 21 Gy in 3 fractions will be optimal in generating an immune response against the tumor. This new trial will address some of the key questions related to safety, efficacy, and the importance of radiating microscopic pleural disease to improve the abscopal effect in mesothelioma. This approach will then provide a platform for immunotherapy.

CLINICS CARE POINTS

- Extrapleural pneumonectomy should be considered for selected patients with mesothelioma, particularly in the presence of diffuse pleural involvement with invasion of the lung parenchyma

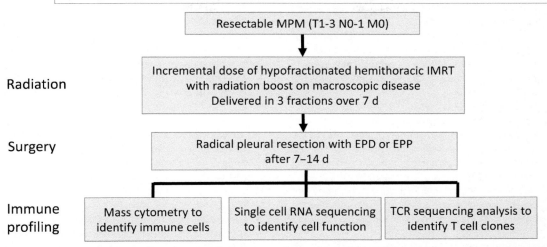

Fig. 6. SMARTER is a phase I clinical trial with increasing doses of nonablative oligofractionated hemithoracic radiation to the pleural space delivered in 3 fractions over 1 week (NCT04028570). This approach will provide a platform for immunotherapy in early-stage mesothelioma.

- Thorough staging workup and physiologic investigations should be performed before extrapleural pneumonectomy
- Meticulous surgical technique and optimal postoperative care must be used to achieve the whole benefit of extrapleural pneumonectomy
- Focus should be on the multimodality approach rather than the type of surgery as long as a complete MCR is performed and multimodality therapy scan be safely delivered
- Nonablative oligofractionated radiation combined with macroscopic complete resection could offer an optimal platform for immunotherapy in early-stage mesothelioma

ACKNOWLEDGMENTS

This work is supported by the Princess Margaret Cancer Foundation and the Toronto General & Western Hospital Foundation.

DISCLOSURE

Marc de Perrot received consulting fees from Astra-Zeneca and Bayer Pharmaceuticals.

REFERENCES

1. Carbone M, Adusumilli PS, Alexander HR Jr, et al. Mesothelioma: scientific clues for prevention, diagnosis, and therapy. CA Cancer J Clin 2019; 69(5):402–29.
2. Zalcman G, Mazieres J, Margery J, et al. Bevacizumab for newly diagnosed pleural mesothelioma in the Mesothelioma Avastin Cisplatin Pemetrexed Study (MAPS): a randomised, controlled, open-label, phase 3 trial. Lancet 2016;387(10026):1405–14.
3. Grosso F, Steele N, Novello S, et al. Nintedanib plus pemetrexed/cisplatin in patients with malignant pleural mesothelioma: phase II results from the randomized, placebo-controlled LUME-meso trial. J Clin Oncol 2017;35(31):3591–600.
4. van Meerbeeck JP, Gaafar R, Manegold C, et al. Randomized phase III study of cisplatin with or without raltitrexed in patients with malignant pleural mesothelioma: an intergroup study of the European Organisation for Research and Treatment of Cancer Lung Cancer Group and the National Cancer Institute of Canada. J Clin Oncol 2005;23(28):6881–9.
5. Vogelzang NJ, Rusthoven JJ, Symanowski J, et al. Phase III study of pemetrexed in combination with cisplatin versus cisplatin alone in patients with malignant pleural mesothelioma. J Clin Oncol 2003; 21(14):2636–44.
6. Churg A, Galateau-Salle F, Roden AC, et al. Malignant mesothelioma in situ: morphologic features and clinical outcome. Mod Pathol 2020;33(2): 297–302.
7. de Gooijer CJ, Borm FJ, Scherpereel A, et al. Immunotherapy in malignant pleural mesothelioma. Front Oncol 2020;10:187.

8. Maio M, Scherpereel A, Calabrò L, et al. Tremelimu-mab as second-line or third-line treatment in relapsed malignant mesothelioma (DETERMINE): a multicentre, international, randomised, double-blind, placebo-controlled phase 2b trial. Lancet Oncol 2017;18(9):1261–73.

9. Calabrò L, Morra A, Giannarelli D, et al. Tremelimu-mab combined with durvalumab in patients with mesothelioma (NIBIT-MESO-1): an open-label, non-randomised, phase 2 study. Lancet Respir Med 2018;6(6):451–60.

10. Scherpereel A, Mazieres J, Greillier L, et al. Nivolu-mab or nivolumab plus ipilimumab in patients with relapsed malignant pleural mesothelioma (IFCT-1501 MAPS2): a multicentre, open-label, rando-mised, non-comparative, phase 2 trial. Lancet Oncol 2019;20(2):239–53.

11. Nowak AK, Robinson BW, Lake RA. Synergy be-tween chemotherapy and immunotherapy in the treatment of established murine solid tumors. Can-cer Res 2003;63(15):4490–6.

12. Wu L, de Perrot M. Radio-immunotherapy and chemo-immunotherapy as a novel treatment para-digm in malignant pleural mesothelioma. Transl Lung Cancer Res 2017;6(3):325–34.

13. Rusch VW, Giroux D, Kennedy C, et al. Initial anal-ysis of the international association for the study of lung cancer mesothelioma database. J Thorac On-col 2012;7(11):1631–9.

14. Nelson DB, Rice DC, Niu J, et al. Long-term survival outcomes of cancer-directed surgery for malignant pleural mesothelioma: propensity score matching analysis. J Clin Oncol 2017;35(29):3354–62.

15. Rusch V, Baldini EH, Bueno R, et al. The role of sur-gical cytoreduction in the treatment of malignant pleural mesothelioma: meeting summary of the Inter-national Mesothelioma Interest Group Congress, September 11–14, 2012, Boston, Mass. J Thorac Cardiovasc Surg 2013;145(4):909–10.

16. Kindler HL, Ismaila N, Armato SG 3rd, et al. Treat-ment of malignant pleural mesothelioma: American Society of Clinical Oncology clinical practice guide-line. J Clin Oncol 2018;36(13):1343–73.

17. Domen A, Berzenji L, Hendriks JMH, et al. Extrap-leural pneumonectomy: still indicated? Transl Lung Cancer Res 2018;7(5):550–5.

18. Friedberg JS, Culligan MJ, Tsao AS, et al. A proposed system toward standardizing surgical-based treatments for malignant pleural mesotheli-oma, from the Joint National Cancer Institute-International Association for the Study of Lung Cancer-Mesothelioma Applied Research Foundation Taskforce. J Thorac Oncol 2019;14(8):1343–53.

19. Burt BM, Richards WG, Lee HS, et al. A phase I trial of surgical resection and intraoperative hyperther-mic cisplatin and gemcitabine for pleural mesotheli-oma. J Thorac Oncol 2018;13(9):1400–9.

20. Burt BM, Cameron RB, Mollberg NM, et al. Malig-nant pleural mesothelioma and the Society of Thoracic Surgeons Database: an analysis of surgi-cal morbidity and mortality. J Thorac Cardiovasc Surg 2014;148(1):30–5.

21. Flores RM, Riedel E, Donington JS, et al. Frequency of use and predictors of cancer-directed surgery in the management of malignant pleural mesothelioma in a community-based (Surveillance, Epidemiology, and End Results [SEER]) population. J Thorac Oncol 2010;5(10):1649–54.

22. Butchart EG, Ashcroft T, Barnsley WC, et al. Pleuro-pneumonectomy in the management of diffuse ma-lignant mesothelioma of the pleura. Experience with 29 patients. Thorax 1976;31(1):15–24.

23. Luckraz H, Rahman M, Patel N, et al. Three decades of experience in the surgical multi-modality manage-ment of pleural mesothelioma. Eur J Cardiothorac Surg 2010;37(3):552–6.

24. Rusch VW, Rosenzweig K, Venkatraman E, et al. A phase II trial of surgical resection and adjuvant high-dose hemithoracic radiation for malignant pleural mesothelioma. J Thorac Cardiovasc Surg 2001;122(4):788–95.

25. Forster KM, Smythe WR, Starkschall G, et al. Inten-sity-modulated radiotherapy following extrapleural pneumonectomy for the treatment of malignant me-sothelioma: clinical implementation. Int J Radiat On-col Biol Phys 2003;55(3):606–16.

26. de Perrot M, Feld R, Cho BC, et al. Trimodality ther-apy with induction chemotherapy followed by ex-trapleural pneumonectomy and adjuvant high-dose hemithoracic radiation for malignant pleural meso-thelioma. J Clin Oncol 2009;27(9):1413–8.

27. Gomez DR, Hong DS, Allen PK, et al. Patterns of fail-ure, toxicity, and survival after extrapleural pneumo-nectomy and hemithoracic intensity-modulated radiation therapy for malignant pleural mesotheli-oma. J Thorac Oncol 2013;8(2):238–45.

28. de Perrot M, Wu L, Wu M, et al. Radiotherapy for the treatment of malignant pleural mesothelioma. Lancet Oncol 2017;18(9):e532–42.

29. Weder W, Stahel RA, Bernhard J, et al. Multicenter trial of neo-adjuvant chemotherapy followed by ex-trapleural pneumonectomy in malignant pleural me-sothelioma. Ann Oncol 2007;18(7):1196–202.

30. Krug LM, Pass HI, Rusch VW, et al. Multicenter phase II trial of neoadjuvant pemetrexed plus cisplatin followed by extrapleural pneumonectomy and radiation for malignant pleural mesothelioma. J Clin Oncol 2009;27:3007–13.

31. Van Schil PE, Baas P, Gaafar R, et al. Trimodality therapy for malignant pleural mesothelioma: results from an EORTC phase II multicentre trial. Eur Respir J 2010;36(6):1362–9.

32. Federico R, Adolfo F, Giuseppe M, et al. Phase II trial of neoadjuvant pemetrexed plus cisplatin followed

by surgery and radiation in the treatment of pleural mesothelioma. BMC Cancer 2013;13:22.

33. Hasegawa S, Okada M, Tanaka F, et al. Trimodality strategy for treating malignant pleural mesothelioma: results of a feasibility study of induction pemetrexed plus cisplatin followed by extrapleural pneumonectomy and postoperative hemithoracic radiation (Japan Mesothelioma Interest Group 0601 Trial). Int J Clin Oncol 2016;21(3):523–30.

34. Frick AE, Nackaerts K, Moons J, et al. Combined modality treatment for malignant pleural mesothelioma: a single-centre long-term survival analysis using extrapleural pneumonectomy. Eur J Cardiothorac Surg 2019;55(5):934–41.

35. Rusch VW, Piantadosi S, Holmes EC. The role of extrapleural pneumonectomy in malignant pleural mesothelioma. A Lung Cancer Study Group trial. J Thorac Cardiovasc Surg 1991;102(1):1–9.

36. Treasure T, Lang-Lazdunski L, Waller D, et al. Extrapleural pneumonectomy versus no extra-pleural pneumonectomy for patients with malignant pleural mesothelioma: clinical outcomes of the Mesothelioma and Radical Surgery (MARS) randomised feasibility study. Lancet Oncol 2011;12:763–72.

37. Weder W, Stahel RA, Baas P, et al. The MARS feasibility trial: conclusions not supported by data. Lancet Oncol 2011;12:1093–4.

38. Cao C, Tian D, Park J, et al. A systematic review and meta-analysis of surgical treatments for malignant pleural mesothelioma. Lung Cancer 2014;83(2): 240–5.

39. Kobayashi M, Ishibashi H, Takasaki C, et al. Pathological evaluation of the visceral pleura in the radical pleurectomy/decortication for malignant pleural mesothelioma patients. J Thorac Dis 2019;11(3): 717–23.

40. Boutin C, Rey F, Gouvernet J, et al. Thoracoscopy in pleural malignant mesothelioma: a prospective study of 188 consecutive patients. Part 2: prognosis and staging. Cancer 1993;72(2):394–404.

41. Rusch VW, Venkatraman E. The importance of surgical staging in the treatment of malignant pleural mesothelioma. J Thorac Cardiovasc Surg 1996;111(4): 815–25.

42. Berger I, Cengel KA, Simone CB 2nd, et al. Lymphangitic carcinomatosis: a common radiographic manifestation of local failure following extended pleurectomy/decortication in patients with malignant pleural mesothelioma. Lung Cancer 2019;132:94–8.

43. de Perrot M, Feld R, Leighl NB, et al. Accelerated hemithoracic radiation followed by extrapleural pneumonectomy for malignant pleural mesothelioma. J Thorac Cardiovasc Surg 2016;151(2): 468–73.

44. Bilecz A, Stockhammer P, Theegarten D, et al. Comparative analysis of prognostic histopathologic parameters in subtypes of epithelioid pleural mesothelioma. Histopathology 2020. https://doi.org/10.1111/his.14105.

45. Quetel L, Meiller C, Assié JB, et al. Genetic alterations of malignant pleural mesothelioma: association with tumor heterogeneity and overall survival. Mol Oncol 2020. https://doi.org/10.1002/1878-0261.12651.

46. Carmichael J, Degraff WG, Gamson J, et al. Radiation sensitivity of human lung cancer cell lines. Eur J Cancer Clin Oncol 1989;25(3):527–34.

47. De La Maza L, Wu M, Wu L, et al. In situ vaccination after accelerated hypofractionated radiation and surgery in a mesothelioma mouse model. Clin Cancer Res 2017;23(18):5502–13.

48. Cho BC, Feld R, Leighl N, et al. A feasibility study evaluating Surgery for Mesothelioma After Radiation Therapy: the "SMART" approach for resectable malignant pleural mesothelioma. J Thorac Oncol 2014;9(3):397–402.

49. Mordant P, McRae K, Cho J, et al. Impact of induction therapy on postoperative outcome after extrapleural pneumonectomy for malignant pleural mesothelioma: does induction-accelerated hemithoracic radiation increase the surgical risk? Eur J Cardiothorac Surg 2016;50(3):433–8.

50. Soldera SV, Kavanagh J, Pintilie M, et al. Systemic therapy use and outcomes after relapse from preoperative radiation and extrapleural pneumonectomy for malignant pleural mesothelioma. Oncologist 2019;24(7):e510–7.

51. de Perrot M, Dong Z, Bradbury P, et al. Impact of tumour thickness on survival after radical radiation and surgery in malignant pleural mesothelioma. Eur Respir J 2017;49(3) [pii:1601428].

52. de Perrot M. Use of the posterior pericardium to cover the bronchial stump after right extrapleural pneumonectomy. Ann Thorac Surg 2013;96(2): 706–8.

53. Vanpouille-Box C, Alard A, Aryankalayil MJ, et al. DNA exonuclease Trex1 regulates radiotherapy-induced tumour immunogenicity. Nat Commun 2017;8:15618.

54. Formenti SC, Rudqvist NP, Golden E, et al. Radiotherapy induces responses of lung cancer to CTLA-4 blockade. Nat Med 2018;24(12):1845–51.

55. Rodríguez-Ruiz ME, Vanpouille-Box C, Melero I, et al. Immunological mechanisms responsible for radiation-induced abscopal effect. Trends Immunol 2018;39(8):644–55.

56. Huang AC, Postow MA, Orlowski RJ, et al. T-Cell invigoration to tumour burden ratio associated with anti-PD-1 response. Nature 2017;545(7652):60–5.

57. de Perrot M, Wu L, Cabanero M, et al. Prognostic influence of tumor microenvironment after hypofractionated radiation and surgery for mesothelioma. J Thorac Cardiovasc Surg 2019;159(5): 2082–91.e1.

Radiation Therapy for Malignant Pleural Mesothelioma

Kenneth E. Rosenzweig, MD

KEYWORDS

- Radiation therapy • Radiotherapy • Intensity-modulated radiation therapy • Mesothelioma
- Pleural IMRT • IMPRINT

KEY POINTS

- Malignant pleural mesothelioma typically presents with disease localized to the hemithorax. Therefore, although distant disease is still a risk, local control is of primary importance after surgical resection.
- Radiation therapy after surgery can reduce the rate of local failure in mesothelioma.
- In most postoperative situations in oncology, the region needing treatment is well-defined, such as a lymph node region or a surgical bed. However, in mesothelioma, the entire pleura is at risk, and this requires a large radiation field that increases the risks of toxicity.
- When administering post-operative radiation therapy after extra-pleural pneumonectomy, the dose to the remaining lung must be minimized.
- After pleurectomy/decortication, because the ipsilateral lung is intact, delivering radiation while sparing the normal lung is technically challenging.

INTRODUCTION

Malignant pleural mesothelioma (MPM) typically presents with disease localized to the hemithorax. Therefore, although distant disease is still a risk, local control is of primary importance after surgical resection. Radiation therapy is a standard adjuvant therapy that is used to improve the rate of local control in a variety of malignancies. In most postoperative situations in oncology, the region needing treatment is well defined, such as a lymph node region or a surgical bed. However, in mesothelioma, the entire pleura is at risk and this requires a large radiation field that increases the risks of toxicity.

Two types of surgery are commonly performed for malignant pleural mesothelioma: extrapleural pneumonectomy (EPP) and pleurectomy/decortication (P/D). EPP involves en bloc resection of the entire pleura, lung and diaphragm, and ipsilateral half of the pericardium. P/D involves resection of all gross tumor without resecting the lung. Although it still has significant toxicity, radiation therapy after EPP is facilitated by the removal of the lung.[1] In fact, part of the rationale for EPP was to allow for the use of high doses of postoperative radiation therapy. In P/D, because the ipsilateral lung is intact, delivering radiation while sparing the normal lung is technically challenging.

Radiation Therapy Techniques

Initially, when administering radiotherapy (RT) as adjuvant therapy following EPP or P/D, patients were treated with conventional radiation techniques using anterior/posterior fields with matching electrons. Local failure with this technique has been reported to be greater than 50% by some centers.[2] Eventually 3-dimensional conformal radiation therapy (3D-CRT) replaced conventional techniques as the standard of care.

Department of Radiation Oncology, Icahn School of Medicine at Mount Sinai, One Gustav L. Levy Place – Box 1236, New York, NY 10029, USA
E-mail address: Kenneth.rosenzweig@mountsinai.org

Thorac Surg Clin 30 (2020) 473–480
https://doi.org/10.1016/j.thorsurg.2020.08.006
1547-4127/20/© 2020 Elsevier Inc. All rights reserved.

Over the past 20 years, intensity-modulated radiation therapy (IMRT) has become a common radiation technique used in many different cancers. IMRT is a highly conformal radiation technique that allows more effective sparing of normal tissues, providing an opportunity for safer, less toxic treatments and increased efficacy by enabling higher radiation doses to the tumor target. It comes with a much higher level of dosimetric control and certainty leads to better target coverage than conventional techniques[3] (**Fig. 1**). A potential disadvantage of IMRT in mesothelioma is dose inhomogeneity and the dose of radiation delivered to the contralateral lung, which potentially leads to a higher risk of pneumonitis.

The National Cancer Database (NCDB) is a large population-based database. An NCDB study compared 3D-CRT and IMRT. It was more likely for IMRT to be used since 2004 and IMRT was also more likely to be delivered at academic centers. However, there did not seem to be a difference in outcome for patients between the 2 techniques.[4]

Another form of radiation therapy is proton beam radiation. Unlike IMRT, which involves the use of photons, protons deposit their radiation energy at the end of their range, known as the Bragg peak. There is a lower entrance dose of radiation

and less radiation delivered along the beam path. Protons have been investigated as a potential treatment of MPM and have favorable dosimetric characteristics. However, because of their high cost of construction, there are currently only 35 proton treatment centers in the United States, and only preliminary work on its utility in MPM has been performed.[5] Protons can be especially useful for patients who have had a local recurrence after prior photon radiation and are in need of reirradiation (**Fig. 2**).

The Role of Radiation Therapy After Surgical Resection

There are limited data with regard to the use of radiation therapy as a standard treatment modality in mesothelioma. A retrospective review of 663 patients from 3 institutions demonstrated improved survival with the use of multimodality therapy as compared with surgery alone.[6]

The role of radiation therapy has been questioned in an analysis of the Surveillance, Epidemiology, and End Result (SEER) database of 14,228 patients with mesothelioma.[7] On multivariable analysis, female gender, younger age, early stage, and treatment with surgery were independent predictors of longer survival. In comparison to no treatment, surgery alone was associated with significant improvement in survival. However, surgery and radiation combined was associated with similar survival as surgery alone. The adjusted hazard ratio for radiation was 1.14 suggesting radiation may not improve outcome in patients with MPM.

There have been multiple analyses of patients in NCDB who underwent definitive surgery for mesothelioma followed by radiation. Nelson and colleagues reported that patients with stage I and II disease who received adjuvant RT had an improved survival. However, this was not demonstrated in patients with stage III or IV disease.[8] A similar analysis by Ohri and colleagues found that younger age, lower comorbidity score, private insurance, surgical resection, and receipt of chemotherapy were associated with increased RT utilization. In addition, patients who received adjuvant RT had higher overall survival at 2 and 5 years.[9] All large database studies, such as SEER and NCDB, must be interpreted with caution due to the lack of detail in a large deidentified database. This is especially relevant in mesothelioma where there is wide variation in the nature of surgical resection and there is no standardization for the RT procedures.

Radiation After Extrapleural Pneumonectomy

Rusch and colleagues[1] at Memorial Sloan-Kettering Cancer Center completed a phase 2 trial

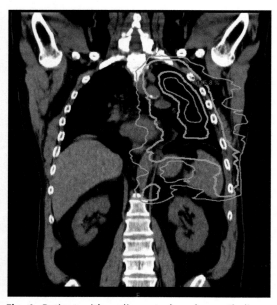

Fig. 1. Patient with malignant pleural mesothelioma after pleurectomy/decortication. Isodose distributions from an intensity-modulated radiation therapy treatment plan in the coronal plane. The 5040 and 2000 cGy isodose curves are represented by the bold green and orange curves respectively. The goal of the plan was to adequate dose to the periphery of the lung while limiting dose to the central portions.

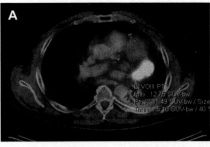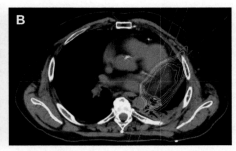

Fig. 2. Patient with recurrent malignant pleural mesothelioma after pleurectomy/decortication and postoperative radiation. Four and a half years after the completion of his initial course of therapy the patient in **Fig. 1** developed a recurrent paramediastinal lesion (*A*). He subsequently received 4 cycles of carboplatin, pemetrexed, and durvalumab with a good response and received 5940 CGE of proton radiation (*B*). One year after the completion of proton radiation he remains disease free.

of EPP followed by postoperative radiation delivered via conventional techniques. Most of the patients (*n* = 62) underwent an EPP followed by 54 Gy. There were 7 postoperative deaths, all primarily related to pulmonary complications in patients who had undergone an EPP. A total of 33 patients had some complications, including atrial arrhythmias, respiratory failure, pneumonia, and empyema. The median survival was 17 months, with an overall survival of 27% at 3 years. Only 13% had locoregional recurrence, with most of the patients who recurred having distant metastases. The investigators concluded that their approach of aggressive surgery with EPP followed by high-dose radiation to the entire hemithorax provided a favorable outcome for those patients who were able to complete the therapy.

Allen and colleagues,[10] from Dana-Farber Cancer Institute, investigated the use of IMRT after EPP and reported a 46% risk of fatal toxicity from radiation pneumonitis. This led many to question the use of this form of radiation therapy. A higher mean lung dose and the volume of lung receiving 5, 10, or 20 Gy have been associated with a greater risk for lung toxicity.[11–13] In the advent of the Dana-Farber experience, further work was done by multiple investigators to establish dosimetric guidelines for the use of IMRT in mesothelioma. Clearly, the dose of radiation to the contralateral (remaining) lung was of primary importance. In the traditional photon-electron technique, the dose of radiation to the remaining lung was minimal because none of the radiation beams were delivered at an angle, which is standard practice for IMRT.

MD Anderson Cancer Center updated their experience in treating MPM with IMRT after EPP.[14] Gomez and colleagues retrospectively analyzed 86 patients who underwent hemithoracic IMRT after EPP. Grade 3 or worse pulmonary

toxicity occurred in 11.6% of patients. Almost all patients had gastrointestinal symptoms, consisting primarily of nausea and esophagitis. There were 5 fatal cases of pulmonary toxicity, 3 from radiation pneumonitis and 2 bronchopleural fistulas. At 2 years, the rates of overall survival, local control, and distant control were 32%, 55%, and 40%, respectively. Fourteen patients (16%) experienced local failure and only 2 of these patients had local failure alone. Fifty-one patients (59%) had distant metastases, which included failures in the contralateral hemithorax and the abdomen.

A review from the University of North Carolina group also examined whether increased experience with received IMRT following EPP led to improvements in outcome.[15] They compared the first 15 patients treated with the second consecutive group of 15 patients. Target coverage (a measure of how well the treatment plan is adequately targeting the tumor) improved in the second group. In addition, the mean dose to the normal structures of the heart and lung also improved in the second group of patients, which suggests that increased experience with this rare disease for the physicians, physics, and therapy staff is of great value in producing high-quality treatment delivery.

A study from the Curie Institute and the Rene Gauducheau Cancer Center, both in France, examined the use of helical tomotherapy (a specialized type of IMRT) after EPP.[16] The investigators used a dose of 50 to 54 Gy with a potential boost to 60 Gy to positive margins. Treatment planning was done to limit the radiation dose to the lung. Twenty-four patients were treated and 4 (16%) had grade 3 or worse radiation pneumonitis within 6 months, including two deaths (8%). There was one case of grade 3 esophagitis. There were only 3 cases of local failure. The remaining patients had distant failure.

An analysis of local failure from the SAKK multi-modality trial revealed that only one patient of 18 eligible patients (5%) had an isolated local failure. Five patients in total had local failure (24%), but the other 4 patients also had a component of distant failure outside of the radiation field. All local failures were in regions that received underdosing of radiation, highlighting the need for consistent and advanced treatment techniques.[17,18]

Radiation Before Extrapleural Pneumonectomy

de Perrot and colleagues[18] from Princess Margaret Hospital reported on an innovative technique to combine radiation therapy and extrapleural pneumonectomy. Patients received 25 to 30 Gy to the entire hemithorax using IMRT 1 week before extrapleural pneumonectomy. Patients with pathologically involved mediastinal lymph nodes received adjuvant chemotherapy. Out of 62 patients, there was only one patient who died in the hospital after EPP and 2 patients who died after discharge for a treatment-related mortality of 5%. Twenty-four patients (39%) developed grade 3 or higher toxicity, which was mostly atrial fibrillation or empyema. No patient underwent radiation therapy without subsequently having surgical resection. The median survival for all patients as an intention-to-treat analysis was an encouraging 36 months. An accompanying editorial suggested that a bold approach such as SMART should only be attempted in centers with significant surgical and radiation oncology expertise.[19]

Most recently, the Princess Margaret group has found that the presence of CD8+ tumor infiltrating lymphocytes was an independent factor for improved survival after SMART, suggesting that the tumor microenvironmental response to radiation may be an important component of tumor control.[20]

Radiation After Pleurectomy/Decortication

With the growing use and potential benefit of P/D instead of EPP,[5] it became an increasing challenge to develop techniques to deliver therapeutic doses of radiation therapy to the entire pleura in the setting of an intact lung. Using conventional treatment planning techniques yielded a 1-year local control rate of 42% and a median survival of 13.5 months.[21] Possible explanations for the poor outcomes include a median radiation dose being only 42.5 Gy and the dose uncertainties with this technique. In addition, the treatment was quite toxic, with 28% grade 3 to 4 toxicity and 2 patients with grade 5 (fatal) toxicity.

Therefore, IMRT was considered to be a potential technique to improve the therapeutic index in these patients. Hemithoracic pleural IMRT (also known as *I*ntensity *M*odulated *P*leural *Rad*iatio*N* Therapy [*IMPRINT*]) has been explored. In this situation, the dose of radiation to the lung as a paired organ would be of dosimetric interest, similar to the challenges seen in the treatment of lung cancer.

Rosenzweig and colleagues[22] from Memorial Sloan-Kettering Cancer Center (MSKCC) reviewed 36 patients treated with pleural IMRT who underwent P/D or biopsy alone. The purpose of the study was to establish the feasibility of pleural IMRT and assess its toxicity. A median dose of 4680 cGy was delivered to the pleural surface and almost 90% of the patients had received chemotherapy, although none received it concurrently. There were 7 patients (20%) with grade 3 or worse toxicity, including one fatality. Five patients (16%) had persistent pneumonitis as a long-term toxicity. The investigators concluded that pleural IMRT is a safe and feasible treatment technique for patients with MPM who have an intact lung on the affected side.

An update of the MSKCC experience evaluated 67 patients with MPM treated with definitive or adjuvant hemithoracic pleural IMRT.[23] Pretreatment imaging, treatment plans, and posttreatment imaging were retrospectively reviewed to determine failure location. Failures were categorized as in-field, marginal, out-of-field, or distant depending on the failures' relation to the 90% and 50% isodose lines. The median follow-up was 24 months from diagnosis, and the median time to in-field local failure from the end of RT was 10 months. Forty-three in-field local failures (64%) were found with a 1- and 2-year actuarial failure rate of 56% and 74%, respectively. For patients who underwent P/D versus those who received a partial pleurectomy or were deemed unresectable (ie, patients who had residual disease), the median time to in-field local failure was 14 months versus 6 months, respectively (P<.03). The investigators concluded that local failure remains the dominant form of failure pattern and that patients treated with adjuvant hemithoracic pleural IMRT after P/D experience a significantly longer time to local and distant failure than patients treated with definitive pleural IMRT.

A retrospective review of all patients who received P/D followed by adjuvant RT was also performed by the investigators at MSKCC. Adjuvant RT was either given conventionally or via IMPRINT. The patients receiving IMPRINT, not surprisingly, had higher rates of chemotherapy treatment. Despite that, on multivariable analysis, the use of IMPRINT had significantly higher overall survival. There was also significant reduction in the rate of grade 2 or higher esophagitis.[24]

Investigators in Aviano, Italy reported on 28 patients who were treated with HT after pleurectomy/decortication or biopsy alone.[25] All patients had FDG-PET scans after surgery for staging and were treated to an intended dose of 50 Gy. Areas that were hypermetabolic on PET were boosted with an additional 10 Gy. The primary pulmonary dosimetric constraint was the contralateral lung to a mean dose of less than 7 Gy. The ipsilateral lung and the total lung did not have specific constraints. Five patients (18%) had respiratory toxicity, but only 2 were grade 3 (7%) and none were grade 5. The percent of contralateral lung receiving 5 Gy was strongly correlated with the risk of pneumonitis. This is especially interesting considering that theoretically there should be some function in the intact lung that might be susceptible to radiation toxicity.

Combined modality therapy

Radiation therapy as part of a multimodality treatment of MPM has been explored. A typical treatment approach has been the use of induction chemotherapy followed by surgical resection and adjuvant radiation therapy. In some of the earlier trials, cisplatin and gemcitabine were used as induction therapy.[26] After a randomized phase III trial established the effectiveness of pemetrexed in combination with cisplatin,[27] subsequent trials explored that chemotherapy regimen before surgery. One multiinstitutional phase II study evaluated 77 patients who received induction pemetrexed and cisplatin.[28] Fifty-four patients subsequently underwent EPP and 40 completed hemithoracic radiation. Median survival in the overall population was 16.8 months. Patients completing all therapy had a median survival of 29.1 months and a 2-year survival rate of 61.2%.

Stahel and colleagues published the results of SAKK 17/04, a multicentered phase II randomized trial. In this trial, patients received 3 cycles of induction chemotherapy with cisplatin and pemetrexed.[29] Patients then received extrapleural pneumonectomy and were subsequently randomized to either hemithoracic radiation therapy or no further treatment. One hundred fifty-three patients were enrolled in the study and 113 underwent surgery. However, only 54 patients went on to randomization. There was no significant difference in local-regional progression-free survival and overall survival between the 2 randomized groups. Although the investigators concluded that there is no role for postoperative radiation therapy after extrapleural pneumonectomy for mesothelioma, it is more likely that this trial was too severely underpowered to detect any difference between the groups.

The use of P/D as the surgical intervention has also been investigated. A multiinstitutional phase II trial of neoadjuvant cisplatin/pemetrexed followed by P/D and IMPRINT is ongoing (ClinicalTrials.gov identifier NCT00715611). The main purpose of this study is to test the feasibility of performing a trial using IMPRINT at various centers, given the complexity of the treatment technique. The NRG cooperative study group has recently opened LU-006. In this trial, patients receive induction chemotherapy followed by P/D. Patients are subsequently randomized to either IMPRINT or no further treatment. This is first phase III randomized trial evaluating radiation therapy in the definitive setting.

Skin boost

Patients with MPM who undergo instrumentation in the chest wall can develop tumor seeding and tumor development at the incision sites. In an effort to reduce the risk of this, prophylactic radiation has frequently been used. It typically consists of a single electron field with a dose of 2100 cGy in 3 fractions. This dose of radiation is not associated with significant side effects.

Boutin and colleagues[30] reported that the use of prophylactic radiation to intervention tracts decreased the risk of subcutaneous tumor development from 40% to 0%. However, a systematic review of the literature showed conflicting results in the multiple trials that had been done.[31] They also reported that there was wide variation in clinical practice in the United Kingdom for this technique.

The group subsequently performed a large multicentered randomized trial of prophylactic radiation versus no radiation. Three hundred seventy-five patients were randomized, and no significant difference was seen in the incidence of chest wall metastases at 6 months between the 2 groups (6% vs 10%). There was a 10% rate of grade 2 and a 0.5% rate of grade 3+ skin toxicity associated with the radiation.[32]

Radiation treatment planning

The determination of the planning target volume and the organs at risk to be avoided is the basis of radiation treatment planning. Given the relative rarity of this disease and the unique aspects of the tumor region, tumor definition can be challenging. An excellent atlas and guide to radiation treatment planning was developed by a joint effort of National Cancer Institute Thoracic Malignancy Steering Committee, the International Association for the Study of Lung Cancer, and the Mesothelioma Applied Research Foundation and should be referenced for physicians who need guidance in caring for mesothelioma patients with radiation therapy.[33]

Similarly to lung cancer, the key organs at risk in treatment planning for mesothelioma are the lungs and the heart. Dose constraints should be developed at each institution due to the individual characteristics of their treatment machines and dose calculation algorithms but should be based on published experience. In general, for treatment after pneumonectomy, the dose to remaining contralateral lung should be kept as low as possible, such as a mean lung dose of 8 Gy or the percentage of lung receiving 20 Gy (V20) less than 7%. These constraints are much lower than typical lung cancer dose recommendations and reflect the fact that there is a single lung and that even a mild radiation pneumonitis can be a fatal complication. For patients with 2 intact lungs, either after P/D or no surgery, a typical constraint is to keep the mean lung dose less than 20 Gy the V20 to 37%. Heart dose may be a significant component of patients diagnosed with radiation pneumonitis. For left-sided tumors a constraint of V40 less than 35% is appropriate. For right-sided tumors, a V40 less than 25% should be used.

SUMMARY

Many aspects of treatment of patients with malignant pleural mesothelioma are still not standardized. There is still variation in the surgical technique used and the role of radiation therapy. The use of pemetrexed chemotherapy is standard, but there is still no clinically effective second-line systemic treatment.

The use of radiation therapy has changed radically since the advent of advanced radiation treatment planning techniques, especially IMRT. IMRT is now part of the care for almost all patients when radiation therapy is used. The publication of the Dana-Farber experience over 10 years ago was a sobering reminder of the potential dangers of new technologies for our patients. Patients with mesothelioma represent an especially difficult population with which to work with because their disease is related to environmental exposures that often leave them prone to other medical comorbidities.

Many thoracic surgeons have decreased their use of EPP in favor of pleurectomy/decortication in an effort to decrease operative morbidity and mortality, especially considering the possibility that there is no clear difference in clinical outcome. Therefore, radiation oncologists will be evaluating patients with 2 intact lungs in need of adjuvant radiation therapy. IMRT, with its ability to deliver concave doses of radiation therapy to complex geometries, is a logical solution to this problem.

The clinical issues for these patients, including contouring, treatment planning, and delivery are not inconsiderable, and it is important to receive care at a center with significant experience in caring for patients with mesothelioma. In addition, although the toxicity for these treatments has decreased, it is not insignificant and must be taken into consideration when treating our patients.

CLINICS CARE POINTS

- Delivering radiation therapy for patients with malignant pleural mesothelioma is technically challenging due to the large anatomic area at risk and the poor health of the typical patient.
- Advanced radiation treatment techniques, such as IMRT or proton beam therapy must radiation must be used to minimize side effects from treatment.
- Special care must be given to minimize radiation dose to the heart and lung(s).
- Prophylactic radiation to sites on the skin where ports had been placed is not routinely recommended.

DISCLOSURE

The author has nothing to disclose.

REFERENCES

1. Rusch VW, Rosenzweig K, Venkatraman E, et al. A phase II trial of surgical resection and adjuvant high-dose hemithoracic radiation for malignant pleural mesothelioma. J Thorac Cardiovasc Surg 2001;122(4):788–95.
2. Yajnik S, Rosenzweig KE, Mychalczak B, et al. Hemithoracic radiation after extrapleural pneumonectomy for malignant pleural mesothelioma. Int J Radiat Oncol Biol Phys 2003;56(5):1319–26.
3. Krayenbuehl J, Oertel S, Davis JB, et al. Combined photon and electron three-dimensional conformal versus intensity-modulated radiotherapy with integrated boost for adjuvant treatment of malignant pleural mesothelioma after pleuropneumonectomy. Int J Radiat Oncol Biol Phys 2007;69(5):1593–9.
4. Shaaban SG, Verma V, Choi JI, et al. Utilization of intensity modulated radiation therapy for malignant pleural mesothelioma in the united states. Clin Lung Cancer 2018;19(5):E685–92.

5. Badiyan SN, Molitoris JK, Zhu M, et al. Proton beam therapy for malignant pleural mesothelioma. Transl Lung Cancer Res 2018;7(2):189–98.
6. Flores RM, Pass HI, Seshan VE, et al. Extrapleural pneumonectomy versus pleurectomy/decortication in the surgical management of malignant pleural mesothelioma: results in 663 patients. J Thorac Cardiovasc Surg 2008;135(3):620–626,e1-3.
7. Taioli E, Wolf AS, Camacho-Rivera M, et al. Determinants of survival in malignant pleural mesothelioma: a surveillance, epidemiology, and end results (SEER) study of 14,228 patients. PLoS One 2015;10(12):e0145039.
8. Nelson DB, Rice DC, Mitchell KG, et al. Defining the role of adjuvant radiotherapy for malignant pleural mesothelioma: a propensity-matched landmark analysis of the National Cancer Database. J Thorac Dis 2019;11(4):1269–78.
9. Ohri N, Taioli E, Liu B, et al. Radiation therapy for localized malignant pleural mesothelioma: a propensity score-matched analysis of the National Cancer Data Base. J Radiat Oncol 2017;6(3):265–72.
10. Allen AM, Czerminska M, Janne PA, et al. Fatal pneumonitis associated with intensity-modulated radiation therapy for mesothelioma. Int J Radiat Oncol Biol Phys 2006;65(3):640–5.
11. Kristensen CA, Nottrup TJ, Berthelsen AK, et al. Pulmonary toxicity following IMRT after extrapleural pneumonectomy for malignant pleural mesothelioma. Radiother Oncol 2009;92(1):96–9.
12. Miles EF, Larrier NA, Kelsey CR, et al. Intensity-modulated radiotherapy for resected mesothelioma: the Duke experience. Int J Radiat Oncol Biol Phys 2008;71(4):1143–50.
13. Rice DC, Smythe WR, Liao Z, et al. Dose-dependent pulmonary toxicity after postoperative intensity-modulated radiotherapy for malignant pleural mesothelioma. Int J Radiat Oncol Biol Phys 2007;69(2):350–7.
14. Gomez DR, Hong DS, Allen PK, et al. Patterns of failure, toxicity, and survival after extrapleural pneumonectomy and hemithoracic intensity-modulated radiation therapy for malignant pleural mesothelioma. J Thorac Oncol 2013;8(2):238–45.
15. Patel PR, Yoo S, Broadwater G, et al. Effect of increasing experience on dosimetric and clinical outcomes in the management of malignant pleural mesothelioma with intensity-modulated radiation therapy. Int J Radiat Oncol Biol Phys 2012;83(1):362–8.
16. Giraud P, Sylvestre A, Zefkili S, et al. Helical tomotherapy for resected malignant pleural mesothelioma: dosimetric evaluation and toxicity. Radiother Oncol 2011;101(2):303–6.
17. Riesterer O, Ciernik IF, Stahel RA, et al. Pattern of failure after adjuvant radiotherapy following extrapleural pneumonectomy of pleural mesothelioma in the SAKK 17/04 trial. Radiother Oncol 2019;138:121–5.
18. de Perrot M, Feld R, Leighl NB, et al. Accelerated hemithoracic radiation followed by extrapleural pneumonectomy for malignant pleural mesothelioma. J Thorac Cardiovasc Surg 2016;151(2):468–75.
19. Rusch VW, Rimner A, Adusumilli PS. SMART or simply bold? J Thorac Cardiovasc Surg 2016;151(2):476–7.
20. de Perrot M, Wu LC, Cabanero M, et al. Prognostic influence of tumor microenvironment after hypofractionated radiation and surgery for mesothelioma. J Thorac Cardiovasc Surg 2020;159(5):2082.
21. Gupta V, Mychalczak B, Krug L, et al. Hemithoracic radiation therapy after pleurectomy/decortication for malignant pleural mesothelioma. Int J Radiat Oncol Biol Phys 2005;63(4):1045–52.
22. Rosenzweig KE, Zauderer MG, Laser B, et al. Pleural intensity-modulated radiotherapy for malignant pleural mesothelioma. Int J Radiat Oncol Biol Phys 2012;83(4):1278–83.
23. Rimner A, Spratt DE, Zauderer MG, et al. Failure patterns after hemithoracic pleural intensity modulated radiation therapy for malignant pleural mesothelioma. Int J Radiat Oncol Biol Phys 2014;90(2):394–401.
24. Shaikh F, Zauderer M, von Reibnitz D, et al. Improved outcomes with modern lung-sparing trimodality therapy in patients with malignant pleural mesothelioma. J Thorac Oncol 2017;12(6):993–1000.
25. Minatel E, Trovo M, Polesel J, et al. Tomotherapy after pleurectomy/decortication or biopsy for malignant pleural mesothelioma allows the delivery of high dose of radiation in patients with intact lung. J Thorac Oncol 2012;7(12):1862–6.
26. Flores RM, Krug LM, Rosenzweig KE, et al. Induction chemotherapy, extrapleural pneumonectomy, and postoperative high-dose radiotherapy for locally advanced malignant pleural mesothelioma: a phase II trial. J Thorac Oncol 2007;1(4):289–95.
27. Vogelzang NJ, Rusthoven JJ, Symanowski J, et al. Phase III study of pemetrexed in combination with cisplatin versus cisplatin alone in patients with malignant pleural mesothelioma. J Clin Oncol 2003;21(14):2636–44.
28. Krug LM, Pass HI, Rusch VW, et al. Multicenter phase II trial of neoadjuvant pemetrexed plus cisplatin followed by extrapleural pneumonectomy and radiation for malignant pleural mesothelioma. J Clin Oncol 2009;27(18):3007–13.
29. Stahel RA, Riesterer O, Xyrafas A, et al. Neoadjuvant chemotherapy and extrapleural pneumonectomy of malignant pleural mesothelioma with or without hemithoracic radiotherapy (SAKK 17/04): a randomised, international, multicentre phase 2 trial. Lancet Oncol 2015;16(16):1651–8.

30. Boutin C, Rey F, Viallat JR. Prevention of malignant seeding after invasive diagnostic procedures in patients with pleural mesothelioma - a randomized trial of local radiotherapy. Chest 1995;108: 754–8.

31. Lee C, Bayman N, Swindell R, et al. Prophylactic radiotherapy to intervention sites in mesothelioma: A systematic review and survey of UK practice. Lung Cancer 2009;66(2):150–6.

32. Bayman N, Appel W, Ashcroft L, et al. Prophylactic irradiation of tracts in patients with malignant pleural mesothelioma: an open-label, multicenter, phase III randomized trial. J Clin Oncol 2019; 37(14):1200.

33. Gomez DR, Rimner A, Simone CB, et al. The use of radiation therapy for the treatment of malignant pleural mesothelioma: expert opinion from the national cancer institute thoracic malignancy steering committee, international association for the study of lung cancer, and mesothelioma applied research foundation. J Thorac Oncol 2019;14(7): 1172–83.

Taken Together
Effective Multimodal Approaches for Malignant Pleural Mesothelioma

Kimberly J. Song, MD[a], Raja M. Flores, MD[a],*, Andrea S. Wolf, MD, MPH[b]

KEYWORDS

- Treatment for malignant pleural mesothelioma • Extrapleural pneumonectomy
- Pleurectomy/decortication • Multimodal therapy in mesothelioma

KEY POINTS

- Multimodal therapy is the preferred approach to patients with malignant pleural mesothelioma and is most likely available at experienced tertiary care centers.
- Although malignant pleural mesothelioma treatment has not yet been standardized, surgical debulking remains the cornerstone of treatment.
- Systemic chemotherapy and radiation therapy remain important adjuncts.
- Advances in radiation and immunotherapy may provide important new options in prolonging survival in patients with malignant pleural mesothelioma.

INTRODUCTION

The diagnosis of malignant pleural mesothelioma (MPM) mandates prompt initiation of an aggressive multidisciplinary treatment strategy to prolong survival in this deadly disease for which median survival without treatment is approximately 7 months.[1] Multimodal therapy for MPM generally requires management at a specialized high-volume center with the resources and experience to facilitate efficient and effective treatment. Options typically include surgery, radiation, chemotherapy, and more recently immunotherapy, with the chosen strategy tailored to each patient. The use of more than 1 modality is preferred to maximize treatment efficacy.

DISCUSSION
Surgery as the Cornerstone

Although there is no defined standard treatment regimen for MPM, cancer-directed surgery is a predictor of longer survival and most studies support surgery as the cornerstone in the context of multimodality therapy.[2,3] Unfortunately, although cancer-directed surgery is offered to more than 40% of MPM patients at large tertiary centers, far fewer patients receive surgery outside of this population, including only 22% of patients with MPM in the Surveillance, Epidemiology, and End Results dataset from 1990 to 2004.[2] Surgery for MPM is centered around the principle of macroscopic resection with adjuvant therapy aimed at microscopic disease. Although the initial surgical evaluation often includes pleural biopsy via video-assisted thoracoscopic surgery, the 2 procedures that have served as the foundation of therapy are extrapleural pneumonectomy (EPP) and extended pleurectomy/decortication (PD). EPP involves en bloc resection of the lung, parietal and visceral pleura, diaphragm, and pericardium, and PD involves resection of all involved surfaces while sparing the lung parenchyma. The exact extent of resection is highly heterogeneous and

a Department of Thoracic Surgery, Mount Sinai Health System, Icahn School of Medicine at Mount Sinai, One Gustave L. Levy Place, Box 1023, New York, NY 10029, USA; b Department of Thoracic Surgery, New York Mesothelioma Program, Mount Sinai Health System, Icahn School of Medicine at Mount Sinai, One Gustave L. Levy Place, Box 1023, New York, NY 10029, USA
* Corresponding author.
E-mail address: Raja.Flores@mountsinai.org

Thorac Surg Clin 30 (2020) 481–487
https://doi.org/10.1016/j.thorsurg.2020.08.002
1547-4127/20/© 2020 Elsevier Inc. All rights reserved.

depends on the extent of disease as well as surgeon preference. Although postoperative outcomes have improved for both of these procedures, they remain relatively morbid with a mortality rate of 2.2% to 7.0%.[4–6]

EPP as treatment for MPM was first described in 1976 by Butchart and colleagues.[7] Their early results saw a 31% perioperative mortality rate, although they acknowledged that many of these deaths might have been prevented with better patient selection, altered surgical techniques, or improved postoperative management.[7] Predictors of prolonged survival include epithelial cell type and negative resection margins,[8] an observation made even in the early work from Butchart and associates.

Although morbidity rates have improved over time, they remain relatively high. In 1 series of 183 patients undergoing EPP with adjuvant chemotherapy and radiation, mortality was 3.8% and morbidity 50% (major and minor complications) with a median survival of 19 months for those surviving the perioperative period.[8] Appropriate patient selection remains paramount and quality of life is an ongoing concern after either debulking procedure. A thorough evaluation of physiologic reserve should be performed, including a full cardiopulmonary workup. Despite the likelihood that EPP is more often performed on candidates with a lower operative risk, PD has been associated with much lower perioperative mortality and possibly increased long-term survival.[5,9] The Mesothelioma and Radical Surgery (MARS) feasibility trial aimed to compare the outcomes of EPP with no surgery, but had several limitations, including a failure to accrue adequate sample size.[10] Few meaningful conclusions can be drawn from its results.

Although universally accepted guidelines do not exist regarding a standard surgical approach to MPM, its aggressive recurrent nature is often cited as a reason to avoid EPP. The majority of recurrences after surgery tend to occur locally[5] and, given the dismal nature of this deadly disease, much of the conversation surrounding the benefits of EPP versus PD has involved the effects on patient quality of life. Impaired self-reported quality of life is prolonged after EPP, and brief improvements in fatigue, dyspnea, and chest pain are short lived, with initial improvements devolving back to baseline by 6 months.[11] There are few existing studies directly comparing quality of life after each procedure. A recent meta-analysis from our institution extracted 659 distinct patients and concluded that quality of life was diminished after either surgery for at least 6 months afterward, but was worse for EPP patients across both physical and social measures.[12] Although the negative impacts of PD seem to be less pronounced,[13–15] findings are heterogeneous and it remains unclear whether postoperative decreases in quality of life fully return to baseline. Unfortunately, most available data assessing quality of life after PD or EPP comes from small, single-center, observational studies. In consideration of these and other similar findings,[16–18] our practice has generally been to opt for PD whenever possible to preserve lung parenchyma, pericardium, and diaphragm and potentially leave patients with greater physiologic reserve to withstand adjuvant treatment and maximal quality of life.[19]

Multimodal Therapy for Malignant Pleural Mesothelioma: Chemotherapy

Systemic chemotherapy in the form of combined pemetrexed and cisplatin remains first-line medical treatment since the results of the Evaluation of Mesothelioma in a Phase III Trial of Pemetrexed with Cisplatin (EMPHACIS), a landmark study comparing results from cisplatin versus cisplatin/pemetrexed in patients with unresectable MPM. The response rate, progression-free survival rate, and overall survival rate were all increased in the combination cisplatin/pemetrexed group.[20] For patients unable to tolerate cisplatin, the use of carboplatin/pemetrexed is a viable option.[21,22] For those unable to receive pemetrexed, the alternative combination of cisplatin with gemcitabine has been supported.[23,24]

For patients presenting with resectable disease, chemotherapy can be given either before or after surgery. A number of studies have established the effectiveness of neoadjuvant chemotherapy in the setting of trimodal treatment. EPP followed by radiation and cisplatin/pemetrexed or carboplatin/gemcitabine have reported median survival rates of 25.5 to 39.4 months.[25,26] The previously mentioned MARS feasibility trial, which aimed to compare outcomes after EPP or chemotherapy alone, suggested no benefit of surgery but had limitations including its small cohort and high perioperative mortality rate.[10]

Current recommendations are limited by the lack of quality data from randomized controlled trials, including any comparing neoadjuvant to adjuvant chemotherapy. A systematic review of 45 studies of multimodal treatment approaches found overall survival after adjuvant chemotherapy ranging from 11.0 to 56.4 months, and disease-free survival ranging from 8.0 to 27.1 months. Overall survival after induction chemotherapy ranged from 8.8 to 35.5 months, although the authors cited limitations owing to limited data regarding completion rates of induction therapy. In 4 prospective studies with predominantly completed trimodal therapy, the median survival was 16.8 to 25.5 months with disease-free survival ranging from 7.6 to 44.0 months.[27]

Included in this analysis was data from several studies involving hyperthermic intraoperative chemotherapy, an immediate form of adjuvant treatment involving the instillation of intrapleural chemotherapy, usually cisplatin, to deliver high doses locally. Early data on hyperthermic intraoperative chemotherapy have been conflicting. Although Sugarbaker and colleagues[28] found evidence of a benefit for select populations, other data indicate more frequent complications and worse survival rates after hyperthermic intraoperative chemotherapy in a trimodality setting involving EPP.[29] A recent study of hyperthermic intraoperative chemotherapy with cisplatin/doxorubicin after PD found a median overall survival of 16.1 months, with a survival of 17.9 months for the epithelioid subtype and 28.2 months for those with a macroscopically complete resection. In this cohort of 71 patients, the 30-day mortality was 1.4% and the 90-day mortality was 2.8%.[30] At this point, stronger evidence is needed to either support or disprove the role of hyperthermic intraoperative chemotherapy in current treatment algorithms.

As surgical treatment trends toward a less radical approach, there is ongoing investigation into the effectiveness of multimodal therapy involving PD rather than EPP. MARS 2 is an ongoing clinical trial (NCT 02040272) currently recruiting to investigate outcomes of PD with platinum-based chemotherapy versus chemotherapy alone. Another ongoing study by the European Organization for Research and Treatment of Cancer (NCT 02436733) aims to compare results from initial PD with adjuvant pemetrexed/cisplatin versus neoadjuvant chemotherapy followed by delayed PD.

Improving Treatment Efficacy with Immunotherapy

Immunotherapy for MPM has made recent advances as a potential means of increasing existing treatment efficacy. Cytotoxic T lymphocyte-associated protein 4 and programmed cell death protein-1 with its associated ligand are checkpoint inhibitors that have shown increasing promise as immunotherapy targets. A recent phase IB study has demonstrated that the programmed cell death protein-1 inhibitor pembrolizumab is reasonably safe and effective in this setting, with fatigue and nausea being the most common adverse effects.

In this cohort of 25 patients who had failed or were unable to receive standard therapy, therapy was given every 2 weeks in an ongoing fashion; 20% had a partial response and 52% had stable disease, with a median duration of stable disease of 5.6 months.[31] Further phase II trials are now underway.

The anti-cytotoxic T lymphocyte-associated protein 4 monoclonal antibody tremelimumab, although initially showing promise in earlier single-center studies,[32,33] was subsequently the subject of the multicenter randomized controlled DETERMINE trial, administered to patients with unresectable pleural or peritoneal mesothelioma who had progressed on systemic treatment. The investigators found no difference in survival between treatment and placebo groups.[34] More recently, a phase II study of tremelimumab with durvalumab, an anti–programmed cell death ligand-1 monoclonal antibody, showed promising results with 63% of patients having disease control.[35]

Interest has also grown with regard to the addition of the vascular endothelial growth factor inhibitor bevacizumab to standard first line treatments. In a large phase III study, Zalcman and colleagues[36] reported improved progression-free and overall survival when bevacizumab was added to pemetrexed/cisplatin, although there were increases in the rate of side effects such as hypertension and thrombotic events. Importantly, a benefit was seen regardless of epithelioid, sarcomatoid, or mixed histology. Currently, bevacizumab is an option for first line therapy according to National Comprehensive Cancer Network guidelines.

Antimesothelin antibodies target the mesothelin cell surface glycoprotein, which is present in a variety of solid tumors, though its expression in sarcomatoid mesotheliomas is limited.[37] A phase II trial of 89 patients receiving the antimesothelin antibody amatuximab for up to 6 cycles in combination with pemetrexed/cisplatin showed a 40% partial response rate with another 51% of patients having stable disease.[38]

Radiation for Malignant Pleural Mesothelioma: Targeting Microscopic Disease in a Large Field

Radiation therapy is a critical adjunct in many cancers to decrease local recurrence, and rates of local recurrence in the ipsilateral hemithorax remain high in MPM.[39] Radiation of the pleura involves the entire ipsilateral hemithorax and although removal of the lung via EPP can facilitate radiation, patients with 1 lung have an associated diminished postoperative physiologic reserve. Common complications of adjuvant radiation include pneumonitis and pericarditis, and although less toxic than previous techniques, intensity modulated radiation therapy (IMRT) can still lead to excess radiation to the contralateral lung.[40]

Currently, no consensus exists regarding standard use of radiation in MPM treatment. Adjuvant low-dose hemithoracic radiation and photodynamic therapy have failed to effectively prolong survival or provide adequate local control.[39,41] Although multimodal therapy improves overall survival over surgery alone,[5] a Surveillance, Epidemiology, and End Results data analysis found no survival difference when surgery with radiation was compared with surgery alone and found an increased adjusted hazard ratio for patients undergoing treatment with just radiation.[42] An analysis of data from the National Cancer Database has suggested improved survival rates with adjuvant radiation,[43] although the information from both databases is inherently heterogeneous.

In a review of 86 patients treated at MD Anderson Cancer Center, Gomez and colleagues[44] reported a 6% rate of fatal lung toxicity in patients receiving IMRT after EPP, with another 6% developing severe radiation pneumonitis. The same group published a follow-up study comparing survival after IMRT after EPP or PD and found no differences in grade 4 to 5 toxicity or time to local or distant recurrence, although the survival rates favored a combination of PD and IMRT.[45]

The use of pleural IMRT alongside the growing surgical trend toward PD has been shown to be safe and effective for the ipsilateral lung, although there remains a significant portion of patients who develop chronic radiation pneumonitis.[46] More recent findings have indicated that treatment with PD and adjuvant hemithoracic pleural IMRT results in longer intervals to both local and distant recurrence compared with those receiving partial pleurectomy or definitive IMRT.[47] A phase II study of patients receiving hemithoracic pleural IMRT after chemotherapy and PD reported no grade 4 or 5 toxicities out of 27 patients who completed intended treatment.[48] The median progression-free survival was 12.4 months and the median overall survival was 23.7 months, with a 2-year overall survival of 59% in patients with resectable disease. When assessed in conjunction with chemotherapy and PD, adjuvant hemithoracic pleural IMRT has been identified as a significant factor for increased overall survival.[49]

Few data are available regarding the effectiveness of induction radiation, with the majority of data and experience centered around radiation after EPP or PD. A feasibility study of the Surgery for Mesothelioma After Radiation Therapy (SMART) approach out of Princess Margaret Cancer Center in Toronto described results from a technique of administering 25 Gy neoadjuvant IMRT over 1 week (with a 5-Gy boost to high-risk areas) followed by EPP within 1 week of completed radiotherapy. Patients with pathologically involved N2 nodes also received adjuvant cisplatin-based chemotherapy within 24 weeks of surgery. They reported promising results, with no 30-day or in-hospital mortalities, no bronchopleural fistulae, and only 1 death from empyema during follow-up.[50]

Their follow-up data, encompassing 62 patients over approximately 6 years, reported a 1.6% perioperative mortality, a 4.8% treatment-related mortality, and a median survival on an intention-to-treat basis of 36 months.[51] The median overall survival in the epithelioid subtypes was 51 months compared with 10 months in biphasic subtypes, suggesting a reevaluation of the role for EPP in certain patients at specialized centers.

SUMMARY

Although much remains to be discovered about the ideal approach to MPM, it is clear that effective treatment is not encompassed by 1 approach, and therapy for disease progression can involve any of these modalities. Whatever treatment approach is decided, it is critical to prioritize quality of life given the deadly nature of this disease.

CLINICS CARE POINTS

- Multimodal discussion and therapy is the preferred approach to patients with MPM, and is most likely available at experienced tertiary referral centers.
- Systemic chemotherapy treatments, most commonly in the form of cisplatin/pemetrexed, can be given in a neoadjuvant or adjuvant setting, and emerging immunotherapy targets can increase their efficacy.
- No standard approach exists regarding radiation therapy for MPM, although ongoing investigations may point to a new role for induction radiation.
- Surgery via en bloc resection remains a critical aspect of treatment, and debulking via PD is growing in favor over EPP.

DISCLOSURE

The authors have nothing to disclose.

REFERENCES

1. Sugarbaker DJ, Wolf AS. Surgery for malignant pleural mesothelioma. Expert Rev Respir Med 2010;4:363–72.
2. Flores RM, Riedel E, Donington JS, et al. Frequency of use and predictors of cancer-directed surgery in the management of malignant pleural mesothelioma in a community-based (Surveillance, Epidemiology, and End Results [SEER]) population. J Thorac Oncol 2010;5:1649–54.
3. Taioli E, Wolf AS, Moline JM, et al. Frequency of surgery in black patients with malignant pleural mesothelioma. Dis Markers 2015;2015:282145.
4. Flores RM. Surgical options in malignant pleural mesothelioma: extrapleural pneumonectomy or pleurectomy/decortication. Semin Thorac Cardiovasc Surg 2009;21:149–53.
5. Flores RM, Pass HI, Seshan VE, et al. Extrapleural pneumonectomy versus pleurectomy/decortication in the surgical management of malignant pleural mesothelioma: results in 663 patients. J Thorac Cardiovasc Surg 2008;135:620–6, 626.e1-3.
6. Wolf AS, Daniel J, Sugarbaker DJ. Surgical techniques for multimodality treatment of malignant pleural mesothelioma: extrapleural pneumonectomy and pleurectomy/decortication. Semin Thorac Cardiovasc Surg 2009;21:132–48.
7. Butchart EG, Ashcroft T, Barnsley WC, et al. Pleuropneumonectomy in the management of diffuse malignant mesothelioma of the pleura. Experience with 29 patients. Thorax 1976;31:15–24.
8. Sugarbaker DJ, Flores RM, Jaklitsch MT, et al. Resection margins, extrapleural nodal status, and cell type determine postoperative long-term survival in trimodality therapy of malignant pleural mesothelioma: results in 183 patients. J Thorac Cardiovasc Surg 1999;117:54–63 [discussion: 63–5].
9. Taioli E, Wolf AS, Flores RM. Meta-analysis of survival after pleurectomy decortication versus extrapleural pneumonectomy in mesothelioma. Ann Thorac Surg 2015;99:472–80.
10. Treasure T, Lang-Lazdunski L, Waller D, et al. Extrapleural pneumonectomy versus no extra-pleural pneumonectomy for patients with malignant pleural mesothelioma: clinical outcomes of the Mesothelioma and Radical Surgery (MARS) randomised feasibility study. Lancet Oncol 2011;12:763–72.
11. Weder W, Stahel RA, Bernhard J, et al. Multicenter trial of neo-adjuvant chemotherapy followed by extrapleural pneumonectomy in malignant pleural mesothelioma. Ann Oncol 2007;18:1196–202.
12. Schwartz RM, Lieberman-Cribbin W, Wolf A, et al. Systematic review of quality of life following pleurectomy decortication and extrapleural pneumonectomy for malignant pleural mesothelioma. BMC Cancer 2018;18:1188.
13. Martin-Ucar AE, Edwards JG, Rengajaran A, et al. Palliative surgical debulking in malignant mesothelioma. Predictors of survival and symptom control. Eur J Cardiothorac Surg 2001;20:1117–21.
14. Tanaka T, Morishita S, Hashimoto M, et al. Physical function and health-related quality of life in patients undergoing surgical treatment for malignant pleural mesothelioma. Support Care Cancer 2017;25:2569–75.
15. Tanaka T, Morishita S, Hashimoto M, et al. Physical function and health-related quality of life in the convalescent phase in surgically treated patients with malignant pleural mesothelioma. Support Care Cancer 2019;27(11):4107–13.
16. Ambrogi V, Mineo D, Gatti A, et al. Symptomatic and quality of life changes after extrapleural pneumonectomy for malignant pleural mesothelioma. J Surg Oncol 2009;100:199–204.
17. Ambrogi V, Baldi A, Schillaci O, et al. Clinical impact of extrapleural pneumonectomy for malignant pleural mesothelioma. Ann Surg Oncol 2012;19:1692–9.
18. Vigneswaran WT, Kircheva DY, Rodrigues AE, et al. Influence of Pleurectomy and Decortication in Health-Related Quality of Life Among Patients with Malignant Pleural Mesothelioma. World J Surg 2018;42:1036–45.
19. Wolf AS, Flores RM. Mesothelioma: live to fight another day. J Thorac Cardiovasc Surg 2018;155:1855–6.
20. Vogelzang NJ, Rusthoven JJ, Symanowski J, et al. Phase III study of pemetrexed in combination with cisplatin versus cisplatin alone in patients with malignant pleural mesothelioma. J Clin Oncol 2003;21:2636–44.
21. Castagneto B, Botta M, Aitini E, et al. Phase II study of pemetrexed in combination with carboplatin in patients with malignant pleural mesothelioma (MPM). Ann Oncol 2008;19:370–3.
22. Santoro A, O'Brien ME, Stahel RA, et al. Pemetrexed plus cisplatin or pemetrexed plus carboplatin for chemonaive patients with malignant pleural mesothelioma: results of the International Expanded Access Program. J Thorac Oncol 2008;3:756–63.
23. Favaretto AG, Aversa SM, Paccagnella A, et al. Gemcitabine combined with carboplatin in patients with malignant pleural mesothelioma: a multicentric phase II study. Cancer 2003;97:2791–7.
24. Nowak AK, Byrne MJ, Williamson R, et al. A multicentre phase II study of cisplatin and gemcitabine for malignant mesothelioma. Br J Cancer 2002;87:491–6.
25. Rea F, Marulli G, Bortolotti L, et al. Induction chemotherapy, extrapleural pneumonectomy (EPP) and adjuvant hemi-thoracic radiation in malignant pleural mesothelioma (MPM): feasibility and results. Lung Cancer 2007;57:89–95.

26. Yamanaka T, Tanaka F, Hasegawa S, et al. A feasibility study of induction pemetrexed plus cisplatin followed by extrapleural pneumonectomy and postoperative hemithoracic radiation for malignant pleural mesothelioma. Jpn J Clin Oncol 2009; 39:186–8.

27. Marulli G, Faccioli E, Bellini A, et al. Induction chemotherapy vs post-operative adjuvant therapy for malignant pleural mesothelioma. Expert Rev Respir Med 2017;11:649–60.

28. Sugarbaker DJ, Gill RR, Yeap BY, et al. Hyperthermic intraoperative pleural cisplatin chemotherapy extends interval to recurrence and survival among low-risk patients with malignant pleural mesothelioma undergoing surgical macroscopic complete resection. J Thorac Cardiovasc Surg 2013;145: 955–63.

29. van Sandick JW, Kappers I, Baas P, et al. Surgical treatment in the management of malignant pleural mesothelioma: a single institution's experience. Ann Surg Oncol 2008;15:1757–64.

30. Klotz LV, Lindner M, Eichhorn ME, et al. Pleurectomy/decortication and hyperthermic intrathoracic chemoperfusion using cisplatin and doxorubicin for malignant pleural mesothelioma. J Thorac Dis 2019;11: 1963–72.

31. Alley EW, Lopez J, Santoro A, et al. Clinical safety and activity of pembrolizumab in patients with malignant pleural mesothelioma (KEYNOTE-028): preliminary results from a non-randomised, open-label, phase 1b trial. Lancet Oncol 2017;18: 623–30.

32. Calabro L, Morra A, Fonsatti E, et al. Tremelimumab for patients with chemotherapy-resistant advanced malignant mesothelioma: an open-label, single-arm, phase 2 trial. Lancet Oncol 2013;14:1104–11.

33. Calabro L, Morra A, Fonsatti E, et al. Efficacy and safety of an intensified schedule of tremelimumab for chemotherapy-resistant malignant mesothelioma: an open-label, single-arm, phase 2 study. Lancet Respir Med 2015;3:301–9.

34. Maio M, Scherpereel A, Calabro L, et al. Tremelimumab as second-line or third-line treatment in relapsed malignant mesothelioma (DETERMINE): a multicentre, international, randomised, double-blind, placebo-controlled phase 2b trial. Lancet Oncol 2017;18:1261–73.

35. Calabro L, Morra A, Giannarelli D, et al. Tremelimumab combined with durvalumab in patients with mesothelioma (NIBIT-MESO-1): an open-label, non-randomised, phase 2 study. Lancet Respir Med 2018;6:451–60.

36. Zalcman G, Mazieres J, Margery J, et al. Bevacizumab for newly diagnosed pleural mesothelioma in the Mesothelioma Avastin Cisplatin Pemetrexed Study (MAPS): a randomised, controlled, open-label, phase 3 trial. Lancet 2016;387:1405–14.

37. Hassan R, Thomas A, Alewine C, et al. Mesothelin immunotherapy for cancer: ready for prime time? J Clin Oncol 2016;34:4171–9.

38. Hassan R, Kindler HL, Jahan T, et al. Phase II clinical trial of amatuximab, a chimeric antimesothelin antibody with pemetrexed and cisplatin in advanced unresectable pleural mesothelioma. Clin Cancer Res 2014;20:5927–36.

39. Baldini EH, Recht A, Strauss GM, et al. Patterns of failure after trimodality therapy for malignant pleural mesothelioma. Ann Thorac Surg 1997;63:334–8.

40. Rosenzweig KE. Malignant pleural mesothelioma: adjuvant therapy with radiation therapy. Ann Transl Med 2017;5:242.

41. Pass HI, Temeck BK, Kranda K, et al. Phase III randomized trial of surgery with or without intraoperative photodynamic therapy and postoperative immunochemotherapy for malignant pleural mesothelioma. Ann Surg Oncol 1997;4:628–33.

42. Taioli E, Wolf AS, Camacho-Rivera M, et al. Determinants of survival in malignant pleural mesothelioma: a Surveillance, Epidemiology, and End Results (SEER) study of 14,228 patients. PLoS One 2015; 10:e0145039.

43. Ohri N, Taioli E, Ehsani M, et al. Definitive Radiation Therapy Is Associated With Improved Survival in Non-Metastatic Malignant Pleural Mesothelioma. Int J Radiat Oncol Biol Phys 2016;96:S132–3.

44. Gomez DR, Hong DS, Allen PK, et al. Patterns of failure, toxicity, and survival after extrapleural pneumonectomy and hemithoracic intensity-modulated radiation therapy for malignant pleural mesothelioma. J Thorac Oncol 2013;8: 238–45.

45. Chance WW, Rice DC, Allen PK, et al. Hemithoracic intensity modulated radiation therapy after pleurectomy/decortication for malignant pleural mesothelioma: toxicity, patterns of failure, and a matched survival analysis. Int J Radiat Oncol Biol Phys 2015;91:149–56.

46. Rosenzweig KE, Zauderer MG, Laser B, et al. Pleural intensity-modulated radiotherapy for malignant pleural mesothelioma. Int J Radiat Oncol Biol Phys 2012;83:1278–83.

47. Rimner A, Spratt DE, Zauderer MG, et al. Failure patterns after hemithoracic pleural intensity modulated radiation therapy for malignant pleural mesothelioma. Int J Radiat Oncol Biol Phys 2014;90: 394–401.

48. Rimner A, Zauderer MG, Gomez DR, et al. Phase II Study of Hemithoracic Intensity-Modulated Pleural Radiation Therapy (IMPRINT) As Part of Lung-Sparing Multimodality Therapy in Patients With Malignant Pleural Mesothelioma. J Clin Oncol 2016; 34:2761–8.

49. Shaikh F, Zauderer MG, von Reibnitz D, et al. Improved Outcomes with Modern Lung-Sparing

Trimodality Therapy in Patients with Malignant Pleural Mesothelioma. J Thorac Oncol 2017;12: 993–1000.

50. Cho BC, Feld R, Leighl N, et al. A feasibility study evaluating Surgery for Mesothelioma After Radiation Therapy: the "SMART" approach for resectable malignant pleural mesothelioma. J Thorac Oncol 2014;9:397–402.

51. de Perrot M, Feld R, Leighl NB, et al. Accelerated hemithoracic radiation followed by extrapleural pneumonectomy for malignant pleural mesothelioma. J Thorac Cardiovasc Surg 2016;151:468–73.

![United States Postal Service logo] **UNITED STATES POSTAL SERVICE** ®

Statement of Ownership, Management, and Circulation
(All Periodicals Publications Except Requester Publications)

1. Publication Title	2. Publication Number	3. Filing Date
THORACIC SURGERY CLINICS	013 – 126	9/18/2020

4. Issue Frequency	5. Number of Issues Published Annually	6. Annual Subscription Price
FEB, MAY, AUG, NOV	4	$393.00

7. Complete Mailing Address of Known Office of Publication *(Not printer) (Street, city, county, state, and ZIP+4®)*

ELSEVIER INC.
230 Park Avenue, Suite 800
New York, NY 10169

Contact Person
Malathi Samayan
Telephone *(Include area code)*
91-44-4299-4507

8. Complete Mailing Address of Headquarters or General Business Office of Publisher *(Not printer)*

ELSEVIER INC.
230 Park Avenue, Suite 800
New York, NY 10169

9. Full Names and Complete Mailing Addresses of Publisher, Editor, and Managing Editor *(Do not leave blank)*

Publisher *(Name and complete mailing address)*

Dolores Meloni, ELSEVIER INC.
1600 JOHN F KENNEDY BLVD. SUITE 1800
PHILADELPHIA, PA 19103-2899

Editor *(Name and complete mailing address)*

JOHN VASSALLO, ELSEVIER INC.
1600 JOHN F KENNEDY BLVD. SUITE 1800
PHILADELPHIA, PA 19103-2899

Managing Editor *(Name and complete mailing address)*

PATRICK MANLEY, ELSEVIER INC.
1600 JOHN F KENNEDY BLVD. SUITE 1800
PHILADELPHIA, PA 19103-2899

10. Owner *(Do not leave blank. If the publication is owned by a corporation, give the name and address of the corporation immediately followed by the names and addresses of all stockholders owning or holding 1 percent or more of the total amount of stock. If not owned by a corporation, give the names and addresses of the individual owners. If owned by a partnership or other unincorporated firm, give its name and address as well as those of each individual owner. If the publication is published by a nonprofit organization, give its name and address.)*

Full Name	Complete Mailing Address
WHOLLY OWNED SUBSIDIARY OF REED/ELSEVIER, US HOLDINGS	1600 JOHN F KENNEDY BLVD. SUITE 1800 PHILADELPHIA, PA 19103-2899

11. Known Bondholders, Mortgagees, and Other Security Holders Owning or Holding 1 Percent or More of Total Amount of Bonds, Mortgages, or Other Securities. If none, check box → ☐ None

Full Name	Complete Mailing Address
N/A	

12. Tax Status *(For completion by nonprofit organizations authorized to mail at nonprofit rates) (Check one)*
The purpose, function, and nonprofit status of this organization and the exempt status for federal income tax purposes:
☒ Has Not Changed During Preceding 12 Months
☐ Has Changed During Preceding 12 Months *(Publisher must submit explanation of change with this statement)*

PS Form **3526**, July 2014 [Page 1 of 4 (see instructions page 4)] PSN: 7530-01-000-9931   PRIVACY NOTICE: See our privacy policy on www.usps.com.

---

13. Publication Title	14. Issue Date for Circulation Data Below
THORACIC SURGERY CLINICS	MAY 2020

15. Extent and Nature of Circulation			Average No. Copies Each Issue During Preceding 12 Months	No. Copies of Single Issue Published Nearest to Filing Date
a. Total Number of Copies *(Net press run)*			223	202
b. Paid Circulation *(By Mail and Outside the Mail)*	(1)	Mailed Outside-County Paid Subscriptions Stated on PS Form 3541 *(Include paid distribution above nominal rate, advertiser's proof copies, and exchange copies)*	100	98
	(2)	Mailed In-County Paid Subscriptions Stated on PS Form 3541 *(Include paid distribution above nominal rate, advertiser's proof copies, and exchange copies)*	0	0
	(3)	Paid Distribution Outside the Mails Including Sales Through Dealers and Carriers, Street Vendors, Counter Sales, and Other Paid Distribution Outside USPS®	77	73
	(4)	Paid Distribution by Other Classes of Mail Through the USPS *(e.g., First-Class Mail®)*	0	0
c. Total Paid Distribution *(Sum of 15b (1), (2), (3), and (4))*			177	171
d. Free or Nominal Rate Distribution *(By Mail and Outside the Mail)*	(1)	Free or Nominal Rate Outside-County Copies included on PS Form 3541	27	16
	(2)	Free or Nominal Rate In-County Copies Included on PS Form 3541	0	0
	(3)	Free or Nominal Rate Copies Mailed at Other Classes Through the USPS *(e.g., First-Class Mail)*	0	0
	(4)	Free or Nominal Rate Distribution Outside the Mail *(Carriers or other means)*	0	0
e. Total Free or Nominal Rate Distribution *(Sum of 15d (1), (2), (3) and (4))*			27	16
f. Total Distribution *(Sum of 15c and 15e)*			204	187
g. Copies not Distributed *(See Instructions to Publishers #4 (page #3))*			19	15
h. Total *(Sum of 15f and g)*			223	202
i. Percent Paid *(15c divided by 15f times 100)*			86.76%	91.44%

* If you are claiming electronic copies, go to line 16 on page 3. If you are not claiming electronic copies, skip to line 17 on page 3.

16. Electronic Copy Circulation	Average No. Copies Each Issue During Preceding 12 Months	No. Copies of Single Issue Published Nearest to Filing Date
a. Paid Electronic Copies ▲		
b. Total Paid Print Copies (Line 15c) + Paid Electronic Copies (Line 16a) ▲		
c. Total Print Distribution (Line 15f) + Paid Electronic Copies (Line 16a) ▲		
d. Percent Paid (Both Print & Electronic Copies) (16b divided by 16c × 100) ▲		

☒ I certify that 50% of all my distributed copies (electronic and print) are paid above a nominal price.

17. Publication of Statement of Ownership

☒ If the publication is a general publication, publication of this statement is required. Will be printed   ☐ Publication not required.

in the NOVEMBER 2020 issue of this publication.

18. Signature and Title of Editor, Publisher, Business Manager, or Owner

Malathi Samayan *Malathi Samayan* - Distribution Controller

Date 9/18/2020

I certify that all information furnished on this form is true and complete. I understand that anyone who furnishes false or misleading information on this form or who omits material or information requested on the form may be subject to criminal sanctions (including fines and imprisonment) and/or civil sanctions (including civil penalties).

PS Form **3526**, July 2014 (Page 3 of 4)   PRIVACY NOTICE: See our privacy policy on www.usps.com

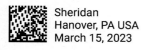

Sheridan
Hanover, PA USA
March 15, 2023